A How To **Self-Help Guide**

Fibromyalgia
and Myofascial Pain Syndrome

A practical guide
to getting on with
your life

Dr Chris Jenner

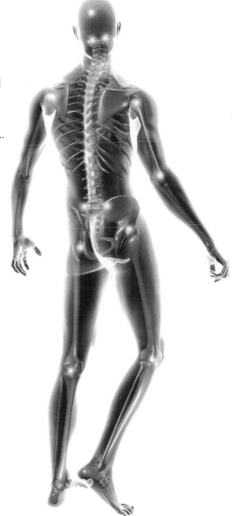

howtobooks

Published by How To Books Ltd
Spring Hill House, Spring Hill Road
Begbroke, Oxford OX5 1RX
Tel: (01865) 375794. Fax: (01865) 379162
info@howtobooks.co.uk
www.howtobooks.co.uk

How To Books greatly reduce the carbon footprint of their books by sourcing
their typesetting and printing in the UK.

British Library Cataloguing in Publication Data
A catalogue record for this book is available from the British Library

ISBN 978 1 84528 467 1

Produced for How To Books by Deer Park Productions, Tavistock
Typeset by PDQ Typesetting Ltd, Newcastle-under-Lyme, Staffs.
Printed and bound in Great Britain by MPG Books Group, Bodmin, Cornwall

NOTE: The material contained in this book is set out in good faith for general
guidance and no liability can be accepted for loss or expense incurred as a result
of relying in particular circumstances or statements made in the book. The laws
and regulations are complex and liable to change, and readers should check the
current position with the relevant authorities before making personal arrangements.

Contents

Part 2: Myofascial Pain Syndrome: Understanding the Basics

Part 3: Living with Fibromyalgia and Myofascial Pain Syndrome

Contents

Part 5: Special Considerations

Preface

Trying to cope with an illness, any illness, is hard enough, but when what you are suffering from is a condition which, even now, some doctors believe to be nothing more than a psychosomatic condition, it can be particularly hard to stomach.

Let me just start then by dispelling any myths about fibromyalgia and myofascial pain syndrome (MPS) and saying quite categorically that they are very, very real. How do I know this? Because having studied for many years in the field of Pain Medicine and worked with sufferers of these and other chronic pain conditions in my roles as consultant in Pain Medicine and Anaesthesia at St Mary's Hospital, London, and as Director of the London Pain Clinic, I have seen first-hand the devastating effects that they have on my patients.

The people who come to see me for diagnosis and treatment, far from suffering from an imaginary illness, are typically wracked with pain and experiencing everything from chronic fatigue to a wide, complex and frightening array of other symptoms which make even the simplest daily tasks feel impossible. Their lives are filled with frustration as their symptoms come and go, leaving them unable to plan even a day into the future. Frequently they report having visited other doctors, only to be met with scepticism or the inability to diagnose or treat their condition, and typically they are amazed at the degree to which a multi-faceted approach to treatment can decrease their levels of pain and increase their overall quality of life.

Despite being so poorly understood, fibromyalgia and MPS are two of the most prevalent illnesses in the world today. The lack of knowledge which surrounds them, however, means that they can often go undiagnosed and untreated for years, during which time both the mental and physical condition of sufferers can deteriorate considerably. The good news, though, is that with the right care, there is much that can be done to help people with these conditions to improve their quality of life dramatically, and the first step towards that is by doing precisely what you are doing now, educating yourself.

Within the covers of this book, what you will find is not a medical textbook, but an easy-to-read and practical guide to fibromyalgia and myofascial pain. My aim is not to blind you with science or confuse you with lots of medical terminology, but rather to take a straightforward and down-to-earth look at what these two conditions are about and how they might affect different aspects of your life, as well as to consider your options and offer support in terms of getting on with your life.

There really is life after being diagnosed with fibromyalgia or MPS ... and yours starts here!

Dr Christopher Jenner MB BS, FCRA
London Pain Clinic

Part One

Fibromyalgia: Understanding the Basics

1

What Is Fibromyalgia?

Anyone seeking an answer to the question 'What is fibromyalgia?' a few years ago would almost certainly have got a very different response than they would now. While some physicians considered it to be a type of depression or other psychological or emotional disorder, others dismissed it as being a total figment of the imagination, or an illness created by lazy people so that they could avoid doing the things they did not want to do. Even today, some of the less well-informed call it 'the invisible disease' and claim that it was invented by those in the psychiatric field for the sole purpose of selling psychiatric drugs. These suggestions, however, are not only wildly inaccurate, but grossly unfair to the millions of sufferers.

Fibromyalgia, or fibromyalgia syndrome (FMS) as it is sometimes called, is an illness which is the subject of much ongoing research. In many ways it is still little understood, but it is a very real and chronic condition nevertheless, and one which is gaining increasing acceptance amongst those in the medical field. Characterised by aches, pains and stiffness which can manifest themselves anywhere in the body, soft tissue tenderness, muscle spasms, severe and persistent fatigue, sleep disturbances and headaches, not to mention sudden and inexplicable memory loss and the inability to think clearly, it can have devastating effects on the daily lives of sufferers, rendering them incapable of carrying out even the simplest of daily tasks that most of us take for granted. While it does not have any visible symptoms, its impact on work, home and family life is frequently anything but invisible.

Many of the difficulties that the medical profession and others have with accepting fibromyalgia as a genuine condition stem from the fact that it is so difficult to diagnose. With a range of symptoms which closely resemble those associated with literally dozens of other conditions, and no single test which can categorically identify it, it cannot be neatly packaged up and labelled. The aches and pains, which are typically experienced at varying levels of intensity, can appear in one part of the body one day, and somewhere completely different the next, making it all too easy for doctors to assume that the symptoms are made up.

A correct diagnosis of fibromyalgia has been known to take years, and even then is often only achieved through a lengthy process of elimination. During this time, the sufferer not only has to live with the painful and frequently disturbing symptoms, but they have to endure the anxiety of not knowing when the next wave will hit them and how severe it will be. As the doctor struggles to identify the problem, they can grow increasingly concerned that the symptoms are all pointing towards some much more serious underlying condition such as multiple sclerosis, although very rarely have patients been found to develop other rheumatic or neurological conditions in addition to fibromyalgia. In many cases, their difficulties are made worse by accusations of hypochondria or a feeling that their illness is not being taken seriously by their physician. In chronic pain, exhausted and yet unable to sleep, and quite often slightly overweight because movement and exercise are so painful, they fear the worst and sometimes sink into depression and anxiety.

Once a correct diagnosis has been made, the bad news is that, as things stand currently, sufferers can expect to face a lifetime of pain and fatigue, which will inevitably take its toll on the quality of life unless appropriate help and treatment is sought. As yet, no definitive cause of fibromyalgia has been identified and so there is no known cure. Looking on the bright side, however, there is no evidence to suggest that it has any effect on normal life expectancy and pain can be effectively managed and minimised through the use of medication and a range of traditional and alternative treatments and therapies, as well as by lifestyle adjustments to address, amongst other things, diet, exercise and stress management.

Accepting a diagnosis of fibromyalgia, understanding how the condition can affect sufferers in a physical, emotional and psychological sense, and learning how to deal with the illness are absolutely key to minimising its effects on everyday life. Throughout this book, you will not only find a great many suggestions which sufferers have found immensely useful in helping them to live with fibromyalgia, but also sections which deal specifically with the impact that it can have on various aspects of life.

2

How Common Is Fibromyalgia and Who Does It Affect?

Fibromyalgia is a common and widespread condition which is believed to affect hundreds of millions of people around the world. Because of difficulties with diagnosis and the fact that many cases almost certainly go unreported, the exact numbers of sufferers cannot easily be established, but here are some of the most commonly quoted rates of incidence for the UK, the USA and the world.

UK Incidence

The prevalence of fibromyalgia in the UK has never been accurately measured and the reported figures are based on estimates derived from US and worldwide statistics. The NHS, who base their estimate on international statistics, however, put the percentage of sufferers in the UK at between 2% and 4.5% of the population. With the population of the UK reported to be a little over 61,414,000 when the figure was calculated (and at the time of writing), this would mean that anywhere between 1.2 million and 2.8 million individuals in the UK could be affected by the condition.

US Incidence

Most of the statistics for the USA show that between 3 and 10 million of the nation's population suffer from fibromyalgia. At the time of writing, the National Fibromyalgia Research Association estimates that somewhere in excess of 6 million Americans are sufferers, and possibly as many as 10 million, which equates to 2–3.2% of the population. The National Pain Foundation, meanwhile, puts the figure at around 2% or 6 million individuals, and the American College of

Rheumatology estimates 3–6 million. The National Women's Health Information Center, which is part of the US Department of Health and Human Services, estimates that the true figure could be as high 8 million.

The highest figure of all to come out of the USA is based on a review of claims records for a national health insurance database. The review, which was conducted by a team of researchers from the University of Utah Department of Family and Environmental Health, identified 2,595 cases of fibromyalgia in a total of 62,000 subjects. This would indicate a rate of incidence of 4.2% which, when applied to the current population in the USA, would put the total number of sufferers at almost 12.9 million.

Global Incidence

The global estimates for the prevalence of fibromyalgia vary hugely, with one source alone quoting anywhere between 0.7% and 4.5% of the world's population being affected. The National Fibromyalgia Association, however, puts the figure at between 3% and 6%, which would account for somewhere between 200 and 400 million people worldwide, based on an estimated global population of 6,816,322,780 in April 2010.

～

Generally speaking, fibromyalgia is no respecter of worldwide location, ethnic origin, gender or age, and cases have been reported in all age groups from children right through to senior citizens. It does, however, have some very significant preferences.

The Gender Issue

Although no explanation can yet be offered as to why, the vast majority of people with fibromyalgia are known to be women, with most sources estimating that females make up between 80% and 90% of the total number of sufferers. These figures seem to be broadly consistent regardless of where in the world the individuals live or originate from, although some research does suggest a higher incidence in African-American women.

Various suggestions have been put forward as to why women are more prone to fibromyalgia than men, and researchers are looking into the role that hormones, differences in the immune systems of men and women, brain chemistry and genetics might play in order to shed some light on this issue.

The Age Issue

The symptoms of fibromyalgia typically appear between the ages of 20 and 55 but, as noted previously, there are also reported cases of the condition appearing in children, adolescents and the elderly. While some studies have indicated a peak in the number of reported cases at around the age of 35, others suggest that symptoms more commonly present themselves between the ages of 40 and 55.

Why Women?

One thing which appears to be significant about the incidence of fibromyalgia in women is that whilst the onset most commonly occurs when they are at child-bearing age, the majority of cases present themselves at middle age. With the average woman beginning menopause at between 40 and 55, some studies have shown a relationship between the declining levels of oestrogen which are experienced at this time and the onset of the condition. In addition, those women who are at the post-menopausal stage often report more severe fibromyalgia symptoms than those who are pre-menopausal, and many of the symptoms which are caused by the significantly lower levels of oestrogen left in the body are common to those of fibromyalgia, including sleep disorders, depression and anxiety.

Another theory concerning hormone levels and fibromyalgia relates to the use of the birth control pill, which of course a greater proportion of women of childbearing age take now than in the past. While some have questioned whether the build-up of the effects of taking high dosage oestrogen pills could actually be a cause of the condition, others have noticed that discontinuing use of the pill has helped to alleviate symptoms such as headaches, muscle cramps and fatigue.

Interestingly, there could also be a link between genes, oestrogen and fibromyalgia. Some research has found that four different gene variants exist in higher levels in individuals who suffer from fibromyalgia, one of which is a variant of the oestrogen-sensitive COMT gene. Perhaps even more significantly, the COMT gene, which the popular press nicknamed 'the pain tolerance gene', has been shown to demonstrate variations which affect people's responses to pain. Scientists in Germany and the United States have also discovered evidence that a variant of the COMT gene may also make some individuals more prone to anxiety disorders, which of course many fibromyalgia sufferers are also more susceptible to.

Fibromyalgia – The Key Symptoms

Fibromyalgia, as we have already mentioned, is notoriously difficult to diagnose, not least because the symptoms are wide-ranging, unique to each individual and highly unpredictable. Many sufferers, however, do experience the majority of the most common symptoms, and these are the ones that we are going to look at in this chapter. In addition to these, however, there are a whole host of other medical problems which are linked to fibromyalgia and are commonly experienced by sufferers of the condition, and these will be considered in Chapter 4.

Musculoskeletal Pain

Widespread and extreme pain, which can affect any of 18 different muscle groups located around the body but is most commonly felt in the neck, back, shoulders, pelvic region and hands, is one of the most classic symptoms of fibromyalgia. Although the pain actually originates from the muscles, tendons and ligaments, sufferers often feel as though it is coming from their joints. Joint pain, however, is known as arthritis, and extensive research has shown that sufferers of fibromyalgia do not have arthritis.

The type of pain that fibromyalgia sufferers experience knows no bounds. It can be an ache which is felt deep inside the muscles, a throbbing pain, a sharp, stabbing pain or even a burning sensation which may feel like severe sunburn. Pain symptoms are quite often worse first thing in the morning and are present even when the sufferer is resting. Generally though, they are more noticeable when the muscles are being used, particularly for repetitive activities.

In their attempts to describe fibromyalgia pain, some have likened it to that experienced during a severe bout of flu, when every muscle in the body feels as though it is in agony. In reality, however, the intensity of the pain does change, so that sometimes it will feel worse than this, and at other times slightly better.

Heightened Sensitivity to Pain

Fibromyalgia, as well as giving rise to widespread and localised pain, can also cause sufferers to experience extreme sensitivity to pain, something which led Swedish researchers Thomas Lundeberg and Irene Lund to ask the question, 'Did "The Princess on the Pea" suffer from fibromyalgia syndrome?' The 'Princess on the Pea' is, of course, the literal translation of the title of Hans Christian Andersen's famous fairy tale which we know as 'The Princess and the Pea', a story in which the main character is declared a princess because of her ability to feel a pea which was placed under 20 mattresses. Not only did the poor woman suffer from a heightened sensitivity to pain, but also from the fatigue and sleep disturbances which are also typical of the condition.

For some people, this increased sensitivity is felt all over the body, to the extent that even the slightest touch is acutely painful. In addition, however, a knock or bump can send pain thresholds through the roof, with the soreness lasting for much longer periods than it would for a non-sufferer.

Although the relatively few specific studies which have taken place to date have shown no conclusive evidence of this, there is also a theory that fibromyalgia patients may suffer from a more generalised sensory amplification, making them more sensitive to touch, sound, heat and electrical stimulation. Certain other things too, such as specific types of food, bright lights and smoke, are also believed to aggravate fibromyalgia symptoms, and sufferers have also been known to experience tinnitus, a condition in which a person has the perception of a noise in one or both ears which comes from inside the body.

Stiffness

Stiffness of the muscles, tendons and ligaments, particularly upon waking, is believed to affect around 90% of fibromyalgia sufferers.

Although the symptom is more commonly felt first thing in the morning, it can also appear after other extended periods of inactivity. Usually it lasts at least 30 minutes up to several hours, but in some cases it carries on throughout the day and into the evening too.

Although morning stiffness can affect any part of the body, the arms, legs, hands, feet and back are normally the most prone. The tightness in the muscles which is typically felt can make it very difficult to sit, stand or rest for any length of time, so even sitting at a desk or taking a short car journey can cause certain areas of the body to feel as though they have seized up. When the symptoms kick in, movement becomes restricted, making it hard for sufferers to go about their normal daily activities, and often the stiffness will be accompanied by a dull, throbbing ache.

Although some say that sleep disorders contribute to the severity of morning stiffness, it is not clear whether sufferers are simply more aware of the stiffness because they keep waking up, or whether they keep waking up because of the stiffness. When a person suffers both sets of symptoms, however, it certainly feels very much like a vicious cycle.

Soft Tissue Tenderness

As well as widespread pain in the muscles, tendons and ligaments, fibromyalgia also causes tenderness in the soft tissues of the body, known as tender points. In response to even the slightest pressure, these tender points generate deep, aching sensations or pain which is described as gnawing, radiating, shooting or burning and can be at either higher or lower levels of intensity.

The tender points which are a characteristic of fibromyalgia are not the same as the trigger points which are seen with other pain syndromes such as myofascial pain syndrome. In the case of tender points, the pain is felt where pressure is applied, whereas trigger points create referred pain in adjacent or distant sites in the body.

Numbness and Tingling

An estimated 25% of fibromyalgia sufferers experience tingling, numbness, a prickling or 'pins and needles' sensation or a burning feeling as part of their range of symptoms. While these can strike any area of the body, including the face, they most commonly affect the arms, legs, hands and feet. The numbness is not necessarily felt throughout an entire limb, however, and might only affect, for example, the area between the shoulder and the elbow or between the knee and the ankle.

As you might imagine, numbness and tingling, particularly in the hands and feet, can have a huge impact on normal daily life. Lifting things can be a challenge, and even walking normally presents the fear of turning, or even spraining or breaking an ankle. Many who experience these symptoms can, quite understandably, also find it impossible to drive, and many different types of work cannot be carried out while the sensations are being experienced.

Fibromyalgia numbness and tingling sensations can appear and disappear suddenly and without warning, and sufferers can often find them frightening because of the fact that these can also be symptoms of other much more serious medical conditions. For this reason, it is important that doctors rule out any other possible causes before making the assumption that the symptom is directly attributable to fibromyalgia.

Muscle Spasms

Like so many of the symptoms of fibromyalgia, muscle spasms can come and go at any time and occur anywhere in the body, although most sufferers complain of muscle contractions in the legs, back and buttocks. In some cases, they might be little more than an annoyance, but in others they can be extremely painful and can make getting a good night's sleep impossible. Quite often, where they appear in the neck, they can lead to a headache which is generally only felt on one side of the head, as well as to feelings of nausea.

Generally speaking, muscle spasms can be caused by a reduced blood flow to the affected area, or when muscles have become overworked, tired and deprived of oxygen. Small tears in the fibres of the muscles can also lead to spasms, as can a deficiency in certain types of vitamins. Again, it is important to rule out other possible causes so that appropriate and effective action can be taken to minimise the effects of muscle spasms.

Cramps

You do not have to have fibromyalgia to appreciate the pain of muscle cramps, but for those who do suffer from the condition the pain can be extreme and long-lasting. Often experienced in the legs and feet, cramps can endure for hours at a time and can severely impact on the ability to sleep.

Although in many cases cramp can feel like a static pain, some have described fibromyalgia cramp as pain which builds and then releases. When experienced, for example, on the inner thighs, this can feel just like the contractions experienced in childbirth, with every bit the same intensity.

Chronic Fatigue

For many fibromyalgia sufferers, chronic fatigue is the most debilitating of all the symptoms. Regardless of how many hours they have slept or of the quality of their sleep, they can feel constantly exhausted and drained of energy. Frequently, they will complain that their limbs feel heavy, making it an effort to stand, let alone move.

Depending on the individual or the nature of the particular 'flare-up', chronic fatigue can be a daily problem or a more occasional one which comes on very suddenly. When it does strike, however, it can make ordinary daily activities such as going to work and doing the housework an extreme challenge, if not impossible. In some cases, people who are experiencing chronic fatigue may even appear to be nodding off whilst in a sitting position, which can make driving or operating machinery particularly hazardous.

Some of the symptoms of fibromyalgia are so similar to those of chronic fatigue syndrome that many believe the two conditions to be linked.

Sleep Disorders

Sleep disorders are another very common symptom of fibromyalgia, with sufferers reporting difficulties in getting to sleep and/or staying asleep. Because what sleep they do manage to achieve does not restore their bodies, they can often wake up feeling completely exhausted. This can be the case even if they appear to have slept for many hours.

Good, regenerative sleep happens in four recognised stages which run from drowsiness and light sleep to the deeper stages of phases 3 and 4. Phase 4, which is the stage when we are in a deep sleep, is particularly important to our bodies because it is then that essential hormones are released which contribute towards the growth and repair of our muscles. Those who suffer from fibromyalgia, however, frequently suffer interruption to phase 4 sleep or do not manage to achieve it in the first place.

What is particularly interesting about sleep disorders is their link to many of the other symptoms of fibromyalgia. Whilst chronic fatigue might be an expected outcome of poor sleep patterns, studies have shown that aches and pains, stiffness and tenderness in the body can all be reproduced by disrupting stage 4 sleep in otherwise healthy subjects.

Alpha EEG Anomaly

Although many consider sleep disorders to be an associated symptom of fibromyalgia, there are those who believe that alpha EEG anomaly could actually be a cause of the condition, simply because such a high proportion of sufferers experience it.

Basically, alpha EEG anomaly occurs when sudden bursts of brain activity happen when the brain should be in deep sleep, something which can be measured on an EEG monitor. While sufferers do not have any difficulty in getting to sleep, when they reach the stage of deep sleep, their brains behave as though they are awake, leaving them feeling drained and exhausted as a result.

Sleep Apnea

Sleep apnea is another very common sleep disorder to affect sufferers of fibromyalgia, and in this case the disorder causes the individual to stop breathing momentarily. While it only happens when the person is asleep, it can affect some so badly that it causes them to wake many times during the night. The gaps in breathing can last for just a few seconds, but in more severe cases they can be as long as a minute.

There are actually two different types of sleep apnea. Obstructive sleep apnea occurs because of a collapse in the airway due to snoring or being overweight, and general sleep apnea, which is much less common, is believed to be caused by a defect in the central nervous system, which essentially means that the brain forgets to tell the lungs to breathe. Although in the first case sufferers may not remember waking up in the night, in the latter they usually do.

In many cases, people who suffer from sleep apnea are not even aware of it and typically it is a partner who notices that they keep waking up. Whilst they might not notice it themselves, however, it clearly still disrupts their sleep patterns and robs them of the essential restorative sleep that they need.

Cognitive/Memory Impairment

Cognitive dysfunction, brain fog and fibro fog are all terms which are used to refer to the state of confusion, poor concentration and sudden and inexplicable short-term memory loss which is commonly reported by sufferers of fibromyalgia. Despite having to deal with extreme amounts of pain as part of their condition, this brain fog is often what sufferers find most disconcerting as it not only leaves them feeling more than a little crazy, but can even be downright dangerous. Feelings of listlessness or lapses in concentration when driving or operating machinery, for example, can lead to tragic consequences.

Some of the most common ways in which brain fog affects fibromyalgia patients include:

- Language difficulties – difficulty in remembering names and common words and the use of incorrect words. These symptoms can make speech sound slow, confused or, in the worst cases, virtually incoherent
- Numerical difficulties – difficulty in remembering numbers, transposing numbers and the inability to do even simple arithmetical calculations
- Short-term memory problems – losing things and forgetting things which have been read or conveyed verbally
- Difficulties in retaining new information – particularly when distracted
- Decreased awareness of surroundings – not being able to recognise familiar places and becoming lost very easily
- Confusion – problems with processing information which would normally be perfectly intelligible
- Concentration lapses – becoming easily distracted or feeling listless and unable to focus one's attention
- Decision-making problems

■ **Problems with multi-tasking – only able to concentrate on one thing at a time**

While the effects of fibro fog might merely be frustrating around the home, in the workplace they can have catastrophic effects as the sufferer may come across as seeming 'under the influence' or incompetent. Because their ability to take in new information can be severely affected, the opportunities for individuals to progress in the workplace, or even to retain a job, can be restricted.

The cognitive impairment experienced by many fibromyalgia patients is also common to sleep disorders which stem from conditions other than fibromyalgia itself.

$\sim$

As you can see, the main symptoms of fibromyalgia can sometimes be so debilitating as to cause sufferers to place severe limitations on their normal activities. Everything feels as though it takes an immense amount of effort and, because patients have no idea how they will feel from one moment or one day to the next, they and those around them commonly feel extreme frustration at the inability to make future plans. Even agreeing to attend a relaxed social gathering with friends in a few days' time can be impossible, without even considering a week-long family holiday.

The physical restrictions placed on sufferers of fibromyalgia can play particular havoc. The pain, stiffness and extreme fatigue that they experience can make any form of exercise feel unbearable, but by avoiding it their bodies become unfit and they frequently gain weight, which only serves to make the symptoms worse.

As we have described, the effects of the condition can also have considerable impact in the workplace. Some individuals may be unable to follow their chosen careers or may have to have their work environment adapted in order to avoid triggering or aggravating their symptoms. Others even have to give up work altogether, although this is something which does need to be considered very carefully. With the potential for the associated decrease in income and loss of self-esteem to provoke stress, stopping work completely can cause the condition to worsen, a subject which we will return to in Chapter 36 which concerns work issues.

4

Related Medical Problems

While the symptoms that we looked at in Chapter 3 could be considered to be the main ones associated with fibromyalgia, there are also a number of other medical problems which are commonly experienced by sufferers, which could be considered to be linked to the condition or which overlap with it. In many cases, individuals might be diagnosed with any one or more of these other medical problems without there being any connection with fibromyalgia, but frequently they do go hand in hand.

Headaches

Headaches, of course, can appear as a single symptom or as part of a whole range of other illnesses, but it is estimated that at least half of fibromyalgia patients suffer from chronic tension headaches which are commonly related to muscle contractions in the head, neck, jaw, shoulders and upper back. In some cases the headache may be quite mild and last only a couple of hours, but often it is severe and can be unrelenting. While some describe the pain as being like a band tightening around their entire head, others find that their temples ache or that the pain is restricted to a specific part of the head, such as the top or only one side.

Alongside all of the other symptoms associated with fibromyalgia, headaches are yet another added burden and they can, in some cases, be quite debilitating in themselves, as well as contributing to feelings of fatigue, depression and anxiety. Although over-the-counter medications can provide some relief, for many people they prove to be largely ineffective. Muscle relaxants and antidepressants frequently offer greater relief, but because fibromyalgia involves such a range of aches and pains, it is often better if prescribed medication is aimed at tackling joint issues rather than individual symptoms. This not only avoids the potential for the overuse of medication, but also the issues associated with side effects and tolerances which are only complicated by taking cocktails of different types of drug.

Migraines

As well as what I will call 'regular' headaches, sufferers of fibromyalgia may also experience migraines. Although many people are inclined to lump migraines in alongside headaches and to think of them as being one and the same thing, any migraine sufferer will fully appreciate that they are, in fact, in no way similar in terms of their characteristics and generally in terms of their intensity.

Migraines come in two forms, the classic migraine and the common migraine. In its common form, it is characterised by extreme pain which is usually felt either to the front or the side of the head and is typically accompanied by nausea, vomiting and/or sensitivity to light. A classic migraine, on the other hand, comes with a warning sign called an aura, which is generally experienced as a visual disturbance such as flashing lights, the impression of 'seeing stars', or blocks of light or patterns which only appear within a certain range of the sufferer's vision. In addition, they may feel stiffness in the neck, shoulders and limbs. In severe cases, migraines can cause hallucinations, disorientation and confusion and can even cause speech to become unintelligible. A bad migraine can often leave the sufferer feeling exhausted and unwell for several days afterwards.

Migraines can be triggered by a number of different things. Certain types of food such as cheese and chocolate, for example, are common triggers, but bright lights, irregular eating patterns, lack of sleep and stress are also known to set them off. When you bear in mind that one of the suspected triggers or aggravating factors of fibromyalgia is stress, and that most sufferers of the condition experience sleep disorders and are already quite often sensitive to things such as light and certain foodstuffs, it is not hard to see the connection between the two complaints.

Although over-the-counter painkillers such as aspirin, paracetamol and ibuprofen can sometimes help with mild migraines, the more severe and classic ones generally require stronger medications which contain anti-emetics (anti-sickness medicines) or drugs which are intended to stop the effects of serotonin and can only be obtained on prescription.

Irritable Bowel Syndrome

Irritable bowel syndrome (IBS), which has also been known in the past as nervous indigestion, spastic colon, irritable colon and laxative colitis, is a condition which affects the gastrointestinal tract and causes a disturbance in the regulation of the bowel function. The abnormal levels of sensitivity and muscle activity cause symptoms which range from bloating, abdominal pain or discomfort and flatulence, to diarrhoea and/or constipation.

Fibromyalgia and IBS are known to frequently co-exist and some suggest that as many as 70% of fibromyalgia patients have reported symptoms of the condition. Although, as musculoskeletal and gastrointestinal disorders respectively, the two conditions may at first appear to have nothing in common, both do seem to be associated with the perception of pain, while causing no physiological damage to the body. More significantly, however, a number of studies have shown that in both conditions there is an overgrowth of bacteria in the small intestine, which is known as small intestine bacterial overgrowth (SIBO).

Essentially, as our food is digested and passes from the mouth downwards, part of its journey takes it through the small intestine, where it meets with one kind of bacteria, and into the colon, where it meets with another type which exists in far greater numbers. When something happens to interfere with the passage of food from the small intestine into the colon, the usually small number of bacteria in the former multiplies, causing the symptoms mentioned above.

Interestingly, it is not only large numbers of sufferers of IBS and fibromyalgia who have been found to have SIBO, but also people diagnosed with chronic fatigue syndrome, food intolerances and allergies, as well as those who have been prescribed repeated doses of antibiotics. Other experts believe, however, that the common theme is stress, because the onset of IBS, fibromyalgia and chronic fatigue syndrome in particular often occurs in the wake of a stressful event.

In common with fibromyalgia and chronic fatigue syndrome, there is no single diagnostic test which can identify a patient as suffering from IBS. Doctors therefore have to rely on recognising symptoms which are typical of the condition and ruling out other complaints for which there is a definitive test. If diagnosed, medication would normally only be prescribed in more severe cases, with most patients responding well to lifestyle changes and, in particular, adjustments to their diet.

Temporomandibular Joint Dysfunction

Temporomandibular joint dysfunction (TMJD) is a condition which causes pain in the muscles and joints in the face, jaw and neck and can also lead to migraines. The temporomandibular joints are basically the jaw joints which allow us to open and close our mouths and chew from side to side. These joints are stabilised by muscles and ligaments and when the latter become painful and tender, this is what is known as TMJD. Sufferers of TMJD frequently become teeth-grinders, and this too can contribute to the incidence of headaches.

Diagnosis of TMJD in fibromyalgia sufferers is difficult because physicians often cannot tell which condition is causing the symptoms. Some sources do, however, suggest that around 25% of those with fibromyalgia also have TMJD, although around 90% experience some type of facial and jaw pain anyway. More than 10 million people in the USA are believed to suffer from the disorder, with women being more susceptible than men, and those diagnosed with chronic fatigue syndrome also being more likely to experience it.

Again, the reasons why such high numbers of fibromyalgia and chronic fatigue syndrome sufferers also develop TMJD is not known, but if, as some believe, sensitisation of the entire central nervous system turns out to be a factor, then this could provide the missing connection.

Interstitial Cystitis/Painful Bladder Syndrome

As well as irritable bowel syndrome, sufferers of fibromyalgia commonly suffer from interstitial cystitis (IC), a painful inflammation of the bladder which can cause bladder spasms, pain and tenderness or discomfort in the bladder or pelvic area. The symptoms also include greater urgency to urinate and greater frequency of urination, with some sufferers reporting the need to empty their bladders up to 60 times per day. Low bladder capacity and incontinence can also be particularly troublesome issues and many people find that the intensity of pain often alters as the bladder fills and empties.

The term painful bladder syndrome (PBS) was developed to take into account all cases where painful urinary symptoms are present but do not necessarily fall into the strictest definition of interstitial cystitis. As such, it covers all cases of urinary pain which cannot be attributed to other causes, although often patients report that the condition began after a traumatic event. In other cases, the sufferers themselves believe it to be associated with a previous and severe urinary tract infection or their high consumption of fizzy drinks, coffee and/or alcohol.

Sufferers of IC/PBS may experience anything from mild to severe pain, which can sometimes radiate to the lower back or upper legs. In women, the symptoms may fluctuate according to where they are in their menstrual cycle, with ovulation and the time just before the onset of a period commonly seeing a flare-up.

IC and PBS, being another two conditions for which there is no definitive test and no known cause, are also ones which physicians sometimes do not believe exist. Despite this, however, over a million people in the USA are thought to suffer from IC/PBS and as many as 400,000 in the UK, the vast majority of these being women.

Although the symptoms of IC/PBS are classic of urinary tract infections, tests actually show no sign of any infection. Despite negative test results, however, doctors frequently prescribe antibiotics as a precautionary measure, something which can cause the condition to flare up and the symptoms to worsen. In the absence of a test for the conditions, diagnosis of IC/PBS is normally made by determining the presence of bladder and/or pelvic pain accompanied by the more frequent and urgent need to urinate, and the absence of positive test results for other similar conditions.

Premenstrual Syndrome

As fibromyalgia affects both men and women, it would clearly be wrong to include premenstrual syndrome (PMS) as a symptom of the condition. Having said this, however, many female sufferers of the condition do find that premenstrual syndrome symptoms worsen after they have developed fibromyalgia. Headaches, back pain, abdominal cramps and insomnia all appear to be more severe, and levels of mental confusion and emotional upset also seem to increase.

Because fibromyalgia sufferers appear to be more sensitive to pain and the condition itself seems to amplify pain, the most logical connection between this and PMS is simply that any existing symptoms are intensified rather than being caused by the illness.

Vitamin E and vitamin B6, as well as calcium, magnesium and manganese have all been found to help with the reduction of PMS symptoms generally.

Heat/Cold Intolerance

As well as the many other types of sensitivities which plague fibromyalgia sufferers, intolerance to heat and/or cold is also a problem for most, although cold sensitivity seems to be the most common. When people all around them are dressed in short-sleeved T-shirts and shorts, they can find themselves feeling icy cold, with hands and feet often being affected worst. For some, feelings of extreme cold can be a precursor to a severe attack of pain. At other times, and frequently at night, they can experience symptoms which are sometimes described as being similar to the hot flushes which accompany the menopause, with profuse sweating commonly being reported. In many cases, patients complain that their body temperature is highly unstable and goes up and down like a yo-yo. Although the reason for intolerances to heat and cold are not fully understood, it seems quite likely that they are related to the general hypersensitivity which is part and parcel of the condition.

Something else which is not uncommon for sufferers of fibromyalgia is a body temperature which is permanently either above or below the norm of 37.0C (98.6F). What many find useful is to take and record their temperature at several different times of the day, and over the course of several days, to try and establish their own norm, as this can be helpful to know in situations where doctors or hospital staff might be inclined to jump to inaccurate diagnoses based on a reading which looks abnormal.

Apart from the general discomfort of feeling either too hot or too cold, intolerance to temperature can also aggravate fibromyalgia symptoms. Cold typically increases the amount of pain that is experienced, which is hardly surprising when you bear in mind that we have a tendency to tense our muscles at times when we feel cold. Heat, on the other hand, can increase the feelings of intense fatigue.

Something to be wary of in respect to cold sensitivity is that this can be a symptom of hypothyroidism, another condition which can co-exist with fibromyalgia. As the thyroid is responsible for regulating body temperature, any abnormality in thyroid levels could affect how the body responds to external variations in temperature and so it is important for these to be checked on a regular basis.

Restless Leg Syndrome

A number of studies have shown that sufferers of fibromyalgia have a higher than normal incidence of restless leg syndrome (RLS) or Wittmaack-Ekbom's syndrome, a condition which is characterised by an unpleasant sensation in the lower limbs, and sometimes the thighs, arms and torso, which many describe as being like a crawling, itching, burning or aching sensation. Such is the sense of discomfort that sufferers feel an irresistible urge to move the affected body part in order to gain temporary relief. The condition can occur on its own, but is frequently associated with cases of fibromyalgia and myalgic encephalomyelitis (ME).

Restless leg syndrome typically occurs when an individual has been physically inactive for a period of time, whether at rest, sitting throughout a long car journey or flight, lying still before sleep or during sleep. Because the only way that the sensation can be alleviated is through activity, getting up and exercising or stretching can be beneficial, but constantly having to do so in the middle of the night clearly causes huge disruptions to sleep patterns, and those who suffer from the condition commonly rise the next morning feeling chronically tired and drained.

While the cause of restless leg syndrome is not known, there are suggestions of genetic links and there are also certain underlying conditions which are believed to be related, of which iron deficiency is one of the main ones. Certain medications are also known to worsen symptoms and these include antihistamines, which are commonly found in over-the-counter cold remedies, and antidepressants.

Periodic Limb Movement Disorder

Sufferers of restless leg syndrome also often have to cope with periodic limb movement disorder (PLMD). Although sometimes described as being similar to RLS, the limb movements which are associated with PLMD are involuntary and they only happen during sleep.

All of us occasionally experience jerking or muscle spasms as we are dropping off to sleep, and these are quite normal and natural and tend not to occur repeatedly. With PLMD, however, the movements are normally rhythmic, typically happening every 20 to 30 seconds, five times or more every hour and throughout the night during periods of non-rapid eye movement (non-REM) sleep. The big toes, ankles and knees are the areas of the body which are most commonly affected, although some sufferers will also fan their toes or move their hips.

Although sufferers of PLMD are normally unaware of their movements, their sleep is disrupted nevertheless and they can often find it difficult to drop off to sleep and to stay asleep. This can, of course, make for daytimes during which they feel exhausted.

PLMD is not only a problem for the sufferer him or herself. Anyone who shares a bed with somebody who is experiencing these random movements can also find their own sleep severely disrupted as they are kicked or kneed during the night.

Depression

As explained earlier, many in the medical profession believed years ago that fibromyalgia was a depression-like illness in itself. Although this is not the case and fibromyalgia is a physical rather than a psychological disorder, an estimated 30% of sufferers have been found to suffer from depression and/or anxiety as well. While some think that these are related to the deterioration in the sufferer's physical status and his or her inability to live life normally, other research suggests that fibromyalgia and depression are linked through family history and that certain people are vulnerable to both illnesses.

Unlike the feelings that we all experience from time to time of feeling sad and down, depression is a serious medical illness which can get progressively worse if left untreated and can ultimately lead to suicidal thoughts or even suicide itself. The condition can cause many symptoms including:

- Feelings of despair and helplessness
- A lack of interest in normal everyday activities
- Low self-esteem
- Feelings of uselessness and inadequacy
- A lack of motivation
- Intolerance and irritability
- Indecisiveness
- Difficulty in concentrating
- Suicidal thoughts

In addition, depression can be responsible for a range of physical symptoms such as:

- Loss of appetite and resulting weight loss
- Comfort eating and resulting weight gain
- Insomnia and extreme fatigue
- Constipation
- Nausea
- Indigestion

While treating depression or anxiety with antidepressants or anti-anxiety medications makes it easier to cope with fibromyalgia, it will not eradicate or cure it as it is not a psychogenic disorder (a physical disease caused by emotional stress). Psychogenic diseases are ones whereby the mind changes the body's physiology so that parts of the body begin to break down – asthma and ulcers are two of the most common types of psychogenic disease – but fibromyalgia is known not to cause any such damage to the body.

Anxiety

Often experienced in association with depression, anxiety is a feeling of being worried, fearful and apprehensive. While normal levels of anxiety are actually useful to us in that they help us to perform better or respond to potentially dangerous situations appropriately, sometimes, without there necessarily being a specific trigger, the feelings can start to take over our lives. When this happens, sufferers can frequently experience physical symptoms such as increased heart rate, palpitations, dizziness, sweating, shaking, nausea and a whole range of disturbing aches and pains, and these symptoms add to the feelings of anxiety and so perpetuate the problem.

For those diagnosed with fibromyalgia, anxiety commonly starts to show itself within a few months of diagnosis. Fears start to build concerning how the condition is going to affect the rest of their lives from a work and home perspective, and before they know it they are not only suffering from the effects of the anxiety itself, but also their fibromyalgia symptoms have worsened as a direct result.

The list of common symptoms which are either directly caused by fibromyalgia or by related disorders is vast, and this of course makes diagnosis and treatment of the condition extremely difficult. With greater understanding and careful management, however, there is much that can be done to alleviate many of these symptoms so that something closer to a normal existence can be achieved.

5

What Causes Fibromyalgia?

Speculation in terms of the cause of fibromyalgia has been rife over the years and yet despite considerable research, it is still unknown. Not only has the job of the researchers been complicated by the fact that the condition affects men and women of all ages, as well as children, but also because there simply has not been enough evidence to support any one particular theory.

While physical examinations of patients have done nothing to help identify a cause for the condition, no diagnostic test has revealed any real clues either. Central nervous system dysfunction, low hormone levels, physical trauma caused by, for example, whiplash injuries, stress, genetic problems, infections, immune system disorders, environmental factors and sleep disorders could all potentially hold the secret of the cause of fibromyalgia, and hence the cure. In this chapter, therefore, we are going to look at some of the theories which could well turn out to have a bearing on why it happens.

Central Nervous System Dysfunction

One of the most popular theories concerning the cause of fibromyalgia is that it stems from a dysfunction of the central nervous system, which comprises the brain, the spinal cord and the nerves. Changes in the neuroendocrine/neurotransmitter systems cause interference with the way in which pain messages are carried and received throughout the body, so magnifying the feelings of pain in what is known as 'central sensitisation'. What might, therefore, feel like a firm handshake to someone who does not suffer from fibromyalgia, could feel to a sufferer as though their hand is being crushed. Such dysfunction may also explain some of the other symptoms of the condition, including the chronic muscle spasms that many sufferers experience.

Why such changes in the central nervous system might occur in the first place is, in itself, a further point for debate. Some studies suggest that certain individuals may be genetically predisposed, while a good deal of other research draws a link between accidents, stress and infection which cause trauma to the body, and the onset of the illness. In these latter cases, it may be possible that the sudden illness or injury sparks off or triggers a previously undetected physiological problem.

Where injuries to the central nervous system are sustained, these can also interfere with the electrical patterns which represent the brain's activities, known as brainwaves, causing sleep disorders, fibro fog and other symptoms which are typical of fibromyalgia.

Trauma and/or Injury

As we have mentioned, the central nervous system can be relatively easily damaged, and not least by motoring accidents, sports and recreational injuries which involve fractures or head injuries, and surgical procedures. Of all of these types of physical trauma, however, it is the whiplash injuries which are sustained in motor vehicle accidents which are most often reported by fibromyalgia sufferers to be the trigger for the start of their symptoms.

Dr Mark Pellegrino, a physical medicine specialist in Canton, Ohio, who specialises in treating patients with fibromyalgia, carried out an analysis of the records of 2,000 of his own patients who had been diagnosed with the condition and discovered that 65% of them had reported the start of their symptoms following a traumatic event. Of these individuals, 52% had been involved in motoring accidents, with whiplash injuries being the most common type. Thirty-one per cent, meanwhile, had sustained work-related injuries and the remaining 17% had suffered other types of trauma such as sporting or recreational injuries.

Another study, which was conducted by Dr Buskila, Professor of Medicine from Soroka Medical Centre, Beer Sheva in Israel, specifically looked at fibromyalgia patients with trauma to determine whether the condition developed after the traumatic incident. Of the 161 people who had suffered traumatic injuries, 102 of them had sustained a typical whiplash injury and 59 had suffered fractures of the leg. While those with the neck injuries went on to develop fibromyalgia 22% of the time, for those with the leg fractures it was only 2% of the time. Dr Buskila used this study to demonstrate that post-traumatic fibromyalgia is 13 times more likely to occur after a neck injury than after a leg injury. Interestingly, insomnia, fatigue and depression, all of which are common symptoms of fibromyalgia, are also two to three times more common after whiplash injuries than after injuries involving the lower limbs.

At the Fibromyalgia, Chronic Pain and Trauma Conference which was held in Bristol, UK, in May of 2001, however, Dr Buskila did admit that there were potential issues with his study, particularly because most of the tender points which doctors use to diagnose fibromyalgia are clustered around the neck and shoulders, the same place where whiplash injuries would also be felt. It would, therefore, be easy for a patient with such injuries to display the symptoms of fibromyalgia, but not so easy for someone who had suffered injuries to the lower limbs. He also noted during the review of his study at the conference that fibromyalgia had typically developed an average 3.2 months after the traumatic event took place.

In most cases of fibromyalgia which are reported in the wake of a traumatic event, patients typically experience severe and persistent pain which is felt in the neck, shoulders and back. Most of these patients are said not to have experienced any ongoing pain before the event and, even though they may have received medical evaluations and treatment at the time of the event, the severe pain had persisted.

Dr Pellegrino's explanation for how trauma leads to fibromyalgia is that peripheral triggers from the trauma bring about both biochemical and neurological changes, first in the muscle and then in the central nervous system. When this process of change begins, the symptoms might only be limited to the specific area of the body where the injury was sustained, but as it progresses, they become more widespread and pain is felt in unrelated areas. Although researchers are still unable to explain why this chain of events might occur, a great many physicians are in agreement that physical trauma can trigger the onset of the condition.

Chemical and Hormonal Imbalances

Although the significance of chemical and hormonal imbalances in fibromyalgia sufferers is not yet fully understood, many studies have found that these individuals do, in many cases, have levels of the hormones serotonin, noradrenaline (also known as norepinephrine) and dopamine which are lower than those found in the average person.

Without getting too technical, serotonin, noradrenaline and dopamine are all neurotransmitters, or chemical messengers which send signals around the body. Each of these hormones plays a particular role in controlling processes of the body which are known to be affected by fibromyalgia patients. Dopamine, for example, controls mood and behaviour and the way that we learn, while noradrenaline is responsible for determining our responses to stressful situations.

Serotonin, which appears to be particularly significant in terms of fibromyalgia, meanwhile, helps to regulate sleep, digestion, pain, mood and mental clarity. Not only have fibromyalgia sufferers been found to have reduced levels of this hormone in their bodies, but also lowered levels of the amino acid, tryptophan, which is used in the production of serotonin.

One of the key things that serotonin does is to raise the pain threshold so that we feel less pain, and it does this by blocking something known as substance P, a protein and neurotransmitter which is found in the spinal cord and is designed to increase the sensitivity of nerves to pain or heighten our awareness of pain. Some fibromyalgia sufferers, therefore, have low levels of serotonin and correspondingly high levels of substance P.

Interestingly, we also have a great many serotonin receptors in the gastrointestinal tract and these help to stimulate digestion. Where low levels of the hormone exist, therefore, there can be disruption to the digestive system, giving rise to the symptoms of irritable bowel syndrome (IBS).

Another imbalance which may be relevant in terms of finding a cause for fibromyalgia is one which is caused by hypothalamic-pituitary-adrenal (HPA) axis dysfunction. HPA dysfunction has been shown to affect sufferers of both fibromyalgia and chronic fatigue syndrome, and effectively it results in the decreased production of human growth hormone (HGH), dehydroepiandrosterone (DHEA) (a prohormone for the sex steroids which impacts on memory and physical performance), cortisol and other hormones. The cause of the suppression of HPA is commonly attributed to chronic stress, but it is also believed to be aggravated by high levels of pain and poor sleep and to be one of the factors linked to cases of depression.

The Genetic Connection

While the role that genetics might have to play in causing fibromyalgia is not understood, many sufferers only have to look to their own families to become convinced that there is in fact a connection. Indeed, this view is supported by a good deal of research which indicates that the condition is more common amongst siblings, parents and children than it is amongst the general population. In one such study, the risk of developing fibromyalgia was 8.5 times higher among the family members of someone with the condition than among family members of someone with rheumatoid arthritis. Many instances have been reported where fibromyalgia spans several generations, and there are also cases where relatives and relations might not share the actual condition itself, but certain of its symptoms, such as chronic fatigue.

Should fibromyalgia come from a hereditary source, what this would mean is not that individuals were necessarily born with the condition, but that they were born with a predisposition or tendency towards it. This is an important distinction when you bear in mind that although in some instances fibromyalgia develops gradually, in the majority of cases it is believed to be triggered by injury or illness. This is probably better understood if you think in terms of a genetic predisposition as being like a time bomb which is ticking away but needs a trigger to make it go off. For those who experience a sudden onset of fibromyalgia, that trigger could well turn out to be trauma caused by an accident, illness or stress.

As mentioned back in Chapter 2, certain variants of the COMT gene (known as the 'pain tolerance gene') could well point to fibromyalgia being a hereditary condition.

Infections

Certain infectious illnesses, including some viruses, are another possible cause of fibromyalgia, although there are two schools of thought on why this might be the case. As some infections attack the central nervous system, this could cause the production of neurotransmitters to be inhibited so that pain messages are not transmitted as they should be. Infections, however, can in themselves cause trauma and injury to the muscles, as well as affecting blood flow, which may then cause symptoms to develop further into chronic and widespread pain. As yet, however, scientists have been unable to identify any specific infectious agent which might trigger fibromyalgia.

Environmental Factors

Although it is well known that certain environmental factors can play a part in triggering flare-ups and aggravating the symptoms of fibromyalgia, there are those who believe that they may indeed be the very cause of the condition. Anything from air pollutants and the chemicals used in the production and manufacture of consumer goods, to the toxins introduced into our foodstuffs and the prescribed and over-the-counter drugs and medications that we use, have all been blamed for the onset of cases of fibromyalgia.

One study which was conducted by the University of Washington and involved 1,400 individuals, even found that those who drank the local well water on a regular basis during their childhoods were 10 times more likely to develop the condition than those who did not. As many of the wells were known to contain environmental toxins such as pesticide run-off, the researchers reported that there could be a definite link between the two, especially in view of the fact that many believe fibromyalgia to be a disorder of the central nervous system.

Some consider that the tendency for fibromyalgia to run in families has more to do with environmental factors than genetics, as family members are often subjected to the same environmental conditions.

Immune System Disorders

Some scientists believe that fibromyalgia could arise as the result of an immune system disorder, but most dispute this on the basis that the symptoms caused by such disorders tend to manifest themselves through inflammation as well as pain. This, of course, is the case with rheumatoid arthritis. With fibromyalgia, however, there is no detectable damage to the body and no signs of inflammation or swelling.

Sleep Disorders

While there is no doubt that a high percentage of those who suffer from fibromyalgia experience sleep disorders as part of their range of symptoms, there is also a theory which puts them forward as the cause of the condition.

The human body needs sleep in order to repair itself, and in particular to ensure that injured muscles and nerves are repaired. If our sleep is light or interrupted and we find it difficult to reach and maintain stage 4 sleep, the deep restorative sleep during which serotonin and human growth hormone is produced, then not only can chronic fatigue be the result, but also chronic pain. In tests, researchers have actually managed to 'reproduce' the symptoms of fibromyalgia by depriving women of sleep. What is unclear, however, is what proportion of fibromyalgia sufferers experienced sleep disorders prior to developing their other symptoms and being diagnosed with the condition.

Stress

The case put forward by many that stress is the primary cause of fibromyalgia is one which requires a good deal further research. Although, as was described under the heading of 'Chemical and Hormonal Imbalances', some believe that links between stress and hypothalamic-pituitary-adrenal (HPA) axis dysfunction could explain the cause of the condition, how these things all fit together is a matter for some dispute. Indeed, there are those who believe that early and severe stress causes the HPA axis to become permanently hyperactive rather than suppressed, although most of the studies which confirm this have only been conducted on animals.

There could, however, be a logical connection between stress and fibromyalgia via muscle tension and sleep disorders. When we are in a state of high anxiety, we unconsciously tense our muscles and when this is done repeatedly it may cause damage to muscles and nerves. When we are stressed, we also find it difficult to achieve the deep, restorative sleep that our bodies need in order to heal themselves, so any damage incurred by the constant tensing and relaxing of muscles does not have the chance to be repaired. This inability to heal properly could then cause continual and severe pain, and the lack of restful sleep would of course also account for the chronic fatigue which most fibromyalgia sufferers experience.

For all of the different theories that exist on the cause of fibromyalgia, sadly none of the research which has been carried out to date has been able to come up with a single, definitive reason why the condition occurs in such a wide range of people from different countries, backgrounds and age groups. Sadder still, of course, is that until a cause is found, there is little hope of finding a cure. For fibromyalgia sufferers today, therefore, all efforts need to go into managing the pain which is associated with the condition, as well as the diverse range of other symptoms. In this respect, however, there are a great many options which can be explored, and we will look at these further in Part 5 of this book.

6

Diagnosing Fibromyalgia

Diagnosis of fibromyalgia can be an extremely frustrating business for doctors as there is no single blood test or X-ray to confirm its presence or absence in patients. The condition does not cause any detectable damage to the body either, so physicians are presented with a whole collection of primary and secondary symptoms but no real signs that fibromyalgia is the cause.

The symptoms of fibromyalgia are so similar to those experienced with other conditions that it can often take prolonged amounts of time to diagnose it, and diagnosis is also complicated by the fact that sufferers of 'well-established' rheumatic diseases such as rheumatoid arthritis, systemic lupus and Sjogren's syndrome sometimes also have fibromyalgia. With all of these difficulties standing in their way, in some respects it is not hard to see why doctors in the past resigned themselves to a diagnosis of depression or other psychological or emotional disorder, or even put the symptoms down to hypochondria, although extensive psychological tests have since shown that psychological issues are not the underlying cause.

If doctors find the diagnosis of fibromyalgia frustrating, then sufferers find it a hundred times more so. At the same time as facing the physical pain and restrictions imposed by symptoms which range from aching, stiff muscles, cramps, chronic fatigue, tension headaches, migraines, IBS, cold intolerance and restless leg syndrome, to name but a few, they frequently have to deal with the mental and emotional fallout and the extreme fear which comes with the inability of their doctors to diagnose their illness quickly. Their minds run riot, imagining all kinds of incurable and either fatal or totally incapacitating diseases, and with no confirmed diagnosis to work with, there is no possibility of putting together a treatment plan to help alleviate their symptoms. The pain and the fear are simply left to grow.

Diagnosis of fibromyalgia, although it may be slow, is however clearly possible, and normally begins with the detailed noting of the individual's personal and family medical history, including a psychological profile, which might help to indicate other conditions such as:

- Infectious diseases
- Physical injuries
- Muscle weakness
- Rashes
- Recent changes in weight
- Sexual or physical abuse
- Substance or alcohol abuse

In addition, it should take account of any prescribed or over-the-counter medications or preparations that the patient is using, including vitamins or herbal medications, as well as of the nature, location and duration of the symptoms which are currently being experienced. From here a process of elimination can begin.

Because the symptoms of the condition are similar to those in upwards of 40 other disorders, some of which may require entirely different approaches to treatment or management and could potentially be very dangerous if left untreated, it is essential to rule these out first by applying tests which are, in most cases, definitive. Blood tests, X-rays, physical examinations and even MRI scans can, for example, pick up such illnesses as thyroid conditions, multiple sclerosis (MS), rheumatoid arthritis and lupus, although they do not necessarily rule out the possibility that these other conditions are co-existing with fibromyalgia. Even once these other illnesses have been taken into account, the physician will still need to consider whether the symptoms that the patient is experiencing could relate to fibromyalgia.

The Criteria for Diagnosis

In 1990, the American College of Rheumatology (ACR) laid down the criteria for making a diagnosis of fibromyalgia and it is these which are used by physicians today. In order to qualify for such a diagnosis, the patient must:

1. Have been experiencing widespread pain for at least three months in all four quadrants of the body, namely on both sides of the body and both above and below the waist, and
2. Be experiencing pain in at least 11 out of the 18 recognised tender points on the body, which are located at:
   - The right and left side of the back of the neck, directly below the hairline and where the neck muscles are attached to the base of the skull
   - The right and left side of the front of the neck, above the collarbone
   - The right and left side of the neck, just below the collarbone
   - The right and left side of the upper back area, close to where the neck and the shoulder join
   - The right and left side of the spine in the upper back area and between the shoulder blades
   - The inside of both arms where they bend at the elbow
   - The right and left side of the lower back, just below the waist
   - Both sides of the buttocks, below the hip bones
   - Just above the knee on the inside of each leg

These 18 points on the body are, in fact, areas which everyone finds more sensitive, so making it easier to test for the signs of hypersensitivity which are typical of fibromyalgia.

Physical Examination

Clearly, for a doctor to be able to make a diagnosis of fibromyalgia based on these tender points he or she has to carry out a physical examination. This will require him or her to apply a standardised amount of pressure (the equivalent of around 4 kg or sufficient to turn the thumbnail white) to each of the 18 points on the body to test the patient's reaction. Rather than merely causing a feeling of tenderness, the pressure should trigger pain at the point which is being pressed, which some describe as being similar to that experienced when pressing on a bruise. It is important also that the physician checks each of these sites to rule out any signs of swelling, redness or heat in both the joints and the soft tissue which might be indicative of inflammation and therefore suggest a completely different disorder. If certain of the tender points cause no reaction when they are first tested, then the doctor may re-test to make absolutely certain of his or her diagnosis, because these tender points can move and change over time.

In addition to testing the tender points around the body, the physician is also likely to look at the nails, skin, joints, muscles, bones and spine as part of the physical examination in order to rule out conditions such as arthritis, thyroid problems and a variety of other disorders.

Tender Points, Not Trigger Points

When considering the diagnosis of fibromyalgia, it is important to note that what the doctor is looking for are tender points rather than trigger points. The term 'trigger point' is one which is used in the diagnosis of certain other conditions, such as myofascial pain syndrome which can often co-exist with fibromyalgia, but trigger points provoke a different reaction than tender points. Whilst a tender point will cause pain directly to the area to which the pressure is being applied, a trigger point refers pain to other parts of the body.

A Note about Anti-Polymer Antibody (APA) Assay

As we have said, there is, as yet, no single definitive test which can diagnose fibromyalgia, but there is one which claims to be the first laboratory test specifically aimed at diagnosing the condition, the Anti-Polymer Antibody Assay or APA Assay.

In a press release dated 10 February 1999, a New Orleans biotechnology company by the name of Autoimmune Technologies, LLC, announced that scientists had discovered a new antibody in the blood of many fibromyalgia patients and developed a patented blood test which could identify these in fibromyalgia sufferers. The company estimates that the test is effective in half of all cases and that more than 60% of fibromyalgia sufferers who experience severe symptoms could be diagnosed using their APA Assay.

There are, however, several important points to note in relation to this test.

1. The company itself admits that the test is not a definitive one, and that even if anti-polymer antibodies do not show up in the test, this does not necessarily mean that the patient is not suffering from fibromyalgia.

2. The research which led to the discovery of the antibodies that the company believes to be present in fibromyalgia sufferers suggests that the condition is 'associated with an abnormal immune system response in these patients'. As we have seen, however, many theories exist as to the cause of fibromyalgia and none of these have been proven categorically.

3. Anti-polymer antibodies have also been detected in patients with other conditions which are frequently confused with fibromyalgia, such as rheumatoid arthritis, systemic lupus erythematosus and systemic sclerosis/scleroderma, although at much lower levels. As the company itself is still in the process of trying to fully understand the nature of these antibodies and why they are produced, one might have to question the validity or the accuracy of any diagnosis made as the result of the test.

4. At the time of the press release in 1999, the company expected to submit an application to the US Food and Drug Administration for approval of a kit form of the Assay as a diagnostic test. More than 10 years later, the Q&A page of their website indicates that the APA Assay has still not been approved for use as a diagnostic test, despite noting that such approval could come 'within six months to a year after the date of submission' of the application.

5. In its 1999 press release, Autoimmune Technologies states that fibromyalgia is difficult to diagnose and that the process of ruling out other illnesses with similar symptoms can be both time consuming and expensive and that 'until now, there has been no laboratory test to help identify fibromyalgia'. While there is no disputing the cost and time factors involved in ruling out other conditions, however, this is an extremely important part of the diagnostic process. Without doing so, physicians risk misdiagnosing a patient's symptoms altogether and possibly applying inappropriate

treatment, or missing the co-existence of other illnesses with fibro-myalgia itself.

~

In summary, therefore, with so little known about fibromyalgia and its causes, and with so many conflicting theories being put forward, those suffering from symptoms which are characteristic of the condition but which could relate to other disorders, might be better advised to stick with the widely-accepted process of diagnosis recommended by the American College of Rheumatology (ACR).

7

Conditions with Similar Symptoms

As we have seen, diagnosing fibromyalgia is not a straightforward process and can be extremely time consuming. What makes it doubly hard, however, are two issues. First of all, a number of rheumatic diseases such as rheumatoid arthritis, systemic lupus and Sjogren's syndrome, as well as other conditions, can co-exist with fibromyalgia. Secondly, fibromyalgia bears strong similarities to, and shares a number of symptoms with certain other conditions. In some cases this has initially led to individuals being misdiagnosed, although a correct diagnosis has usually followed at a later time. Clearly, if the condition is misdiagnosed, there is the risk that the treatment programme which is recommended may have no impact on the condition, and it may even worsen or aggravate it.

Increasingly, the medical profession is becoming more attuned to the presentation of other illness which are similar to fibromyalgia, but it is also helpful for sufferers themselves to be aware of the differences and similarities between them.

Chronic Fatigue Syndrome

Like fibromyalgia syndrome, chronic fatigue syndrome (CFS), or myalgic encephalomyelitis (ME) as it is also known, is another condition which is, as yet, little understood by the medical profession. Characterised, as the name suggests, mainly by debilitating fatigue, it is quite often found in patients after a physical illness such as a chronic viral infection, in the wake of a psychological or emotional illness such as depression or a period of extreme stress, or following an accident. Some experts believe, however, that it is triggered by certain neurological or genetic abnormalities.

The range of opinions concerning links between chronic fatigue syndrome and fibromyalgia is wide. While there is a (thankfully diminishing) proportion of physicians who do not believe that either are bona fide illnesses, there are also those who think that they are completely separate and distinct conditions or that they are two different names for the same condition. As both syndromes share many of the same symptoms including pain, fatigue, headaches, cognitive and memory impairment and sleep disorders, however, the majority of the medical profession is inclined to agree that fibromyalgia and chronic fatigue syndrome are probably related, although no conclusive evidence exists to support this.

Despite the fact that diagnosis of both complaints can be tricky, the main difference between the two lies in the primary symptoms. In fibromyalgia, widespread pain is the most common and severe factor, whereas in chronic fatigue syndrome it is the unrelenting fatigue, a factor which can lead to the sufferer being forced to remain bedridden for days after only minor physical exertion.

In the UK, symptoms of fatigue normally have to satisfy a number of criteria in order to be diagnosed as chronic fatigue syndrome, such as being persistent and/or recurrent, having a specific onset, being unexplained by other conditions and resulting in substantial decreases in levels of activity. In the USA, meanwhile, the Centers for Disease Control and Prevention (CDC) state that fatigue must have been present for more than six months and be accompanied by a sore throat, enlarged or tender lymph nodes, muscle or joint pain or other signs of systemic illness. Diagnosis of fibromyalgia, on the other hand, is largely reliant on the detection of tender points on certain areas of the body.

Although statistics do vary, it is generally estimated that chronic fatigue syndrome affects around a quarter of a million people in the UK and around a million in the USA.

Myofascial Pain Syndrome

Myofascial pain syndrome (MPS) has much potential to be confused with fibromyalgia and is often found to co-exist with it. MPS is dealt with separately in Part II of this book.

Gulf War Syndrome

Gulf War Syndrome is a condition which has been surrounded by controversy and, in fact, many do not believe it exists at all or they attribute it to stress. The illness came to notoriety in the wake of the 1991 Persian Gulf War when soldiers began to experience an array of symptoms including:

- Chronic fatigue
- Headaches
- Muscle pains
- A variety of what were seen as neurological symptoms such as numbness of the arms
- Memory loss
- Sleep disturbances
- Gastrointestinal problems such as IBS resulting in recurrent diarrhoea and constipation
- Skin rashes
- Unusual hair loss
- Cardiovascular problems
- Upper or lower respiratory problems
- Menstrual disorders
- Anxiety disorders

In some cases, the symptoms were so severe as to require hospitalisation and eventually one in four of the 697,000 veterans who took part in the Gulf War were found to have reported similar signs of illness.

The possibilities for the cause of what has been termed Gulf War Syndrome are numerous and researchers are said to be investigating at least half a dozen of these. Parasite infection caused by the bites of sand flies was one of the suggestions, but most of the soldiers who were tested were found to be negative. Depleted uranium (DU), which is a by-product of the material used to fuel nuclear weapons and which is coated on military vehicles such as tanks to protect them from enemy fire, is another possibility. Although when it is intact, DU poses little danger, its release upon impact is known to be hazardous. Exposure to chemical or biological weapons, nerve gas, pesticides, vaccines and medications and exposure to the smoke from burning oil wells have all been put forward as possible causes for the symptoms too.

Those who argue against the existence of Gulf War Syndrome put forward several reasons why they do not believe it to be directly related to the war itself. The fact that no particular platoon or region showed any increased rate of occurrence, for example, is one issue which has led to their questioning the real reason for such huge numbers of soldiers reporting their strange symptoms. In addition, the *New England Journal of Medicine* raises the point that the rate of symptoms reported to be experienced by Gulf War veterans is not significantly different among military who did not take part. With so many of the symptoms being comparable to those associated with chronic fatigue syndrome and fibromyalgia, sceptics have, not surprisingly, been asking whether there is not in fact another explanation which is being overlooked. Like these other illnesses, the causes and potential cure are unknown at present.

Lyme Disease

Lyme disease is actually a bacterial infection which is caused by the bite of certain infected blood-sucking ticks. The disease was named after a number of children in the town of Old Lyme in Connecticut, USA began experiencing what at first appeared to be the symptoms of rheumatoid arthritis, but later on turned out to be an infection transmitted by ticks.

Typically, there are three stages in the symptoms experienced by sufferers of Lyme disease. If the affected individual is treated with antibiotics during the first stage, however, they would not normally be expected to suffer symptoms related to the later stages.

In stage one, which normally develops between 3 and 30 days after having been bitten, many people present with a skin rash at the site of the tick bite which is described as looking like a bulls-eye and which can extend from 2 up to 30 centimetres in a ring around the bite. Not everyone who is affected will develop a rash though, and in fact more than one in four patients do not, making it very difficult to diagnose in many cases. Irrespective of whether a rash appears though, there is usually a range of other early symptoms, including:

- Fatigue
- Muscle and joint pain and stiffness
- Headaches
- Fever and/or chills

As many people are not even aware of having been bitten in the first place and do not experience the rash, these latter symptoms may be the only ones which are presented when the individual goes to see a doctor.

If the disease is not caught at this first stage, then stage two symptoms will usually develop weeks or even months later as the effects of the bacteria spread throughout the body. In around 60% of untreated cases, joint pain and swelling of the joints will present themselves and in certain of these the individual may also find that they experience other symptoms such as:

- Numbness and pain in the limbs
- Impaired memory, difficulties in concentration and sometimes changes in personality
- Temporary paralysis of the facial muscles

In late-stage Lyme disease, which might not develop until many months or even years after the individual received the bite, the symptoms can affect both the joints and the nervous system and can include:

- Chronic and long-lasting joint pain and swelling
- Memory impairment
- Difficulties in concentrating
- Depression and/or anxiety
- Inflammation of the heart muscle
- Abnormal heart rhythms

As Lyme disease can cause serious, long-term problems which could even result in the sufferer requiring a pacemaker to regulate a slow heart rhythm, a correct diagnosis is imperative. Because many of the symptoms do present similarly to those of fibromyalgia though, and particularly because so many people are unaware of the initial tick bite, the two illnesses do risk being confused.

Arthritis

Although fibromyalgia is often categorised as a condition which is related to arthritis, the latter is actually a disease which causes painful inflammation and swelling in the joints, muscles and tissues of the body which can lead to long-term damage. Fibromyalgia, on the other hand, does not affect the joints or cause any direct physio-logical damage, although it can impact similarly on a sufferer's ability to carry out his or her daily tasks due to pain, stiffness, restricted movement and fatigue.

The most common form of arthritis is osteoarthritis, in which the connective tissue or cartilage in the joints breaks down and causes the bones to rub together. The joints which are most commonly affected are the hands, knees, hips and spine and the result is pain, stiffness and loss of movement. Quite often the joints will be swollen too, but because this is not always the case, and because the pain can come and go in just the same way as with fibromyalgia, the two conditions can sometimes be mistaken for one another, at least until such time as other arthritic symptoms present themselves.

Although there is potential for osteoarthritis to be confused with fibromyalgia, it is the other common form of the disease, rheumatoid arthritis, which causes even greater problems with diagnosis. Like fibromyalgia, rheumatoid arthritis is a chronic condition which affects far greater numbers of women and which normally causes fluc-tuating pain and stiffness which feel worse during flare-ups. The morning stiffness which is typically present in both conditions tends to last longer than it does with osteoarthritis, and in many cases rheu-matoid arthritis is accompanied by the same fatigue and flu-like symptoms as fibromyalgia.

Rheumatoid arthritis usually presents with swelling of the joints, but again this may not become immediately evident.

While the standard examination of the tender points around the body should help doctors to differentiate between fibromyalgia and rheumatoid arthritis, the two conditions can co-exist. Not only does this make diagnosis somewhat of a challenge, but treatment too.

Like fibromyalgia, rheumatoid arthritis, an immune system disorder in which the immune system attacks the body's own tissues, has no known cause, although it has long been suspected that sufferers may have a genetic predisposition to the disease, or that viruses, bacteria or environmental factors may play a part in triggering the condition.

Hypothyroidism

Hypothyroidism is the term used for the condition in which the thyroid gland is underactive and does not produce sufficient thyroid hormones. An insufficient supply of these hormones has the effect of slowing down the body's metabolism, which in turn affects, amongst other things, how much a person weighs and how much they sleep.

The symptoms of hypothyroidism are numerous and range from the physical to the emotional and the psychological. Many, however, are ones which are shared with fibromyalgia, including:

- Excessive tiredness
- Joint and muscle pain and stiffness
- Pressure headaches
- Migraines
- Muscle cramps
- Pins and needles
- Constipation
- Intolerance to heat and/or cold
- Insomnia and unrefreshing sleep
- Cognitive and memory impairment
- Depression and/or anxiety

In addition, hypothyroidism can cause:

- Thinning hair and brittle nails
- Weight gain

- Slowed heart rate
- Dry and/or pale skin
- A hoarse or croaky voice
- Swelling of the thyroid gland

Although there are tests for hypothyroidism, in the early stages of the condition the level of thyroid hormones can still be within the normal range, and so doctors do, on occasion, rule it out as a possibility without repeating the test in the future. Instead they might opt for a diagnosis of menopausal symptoms, PMS, depression, stress, chronic fatigue syndrome or fibromyalgia.

8

Fibromyalgia – The Aggravating Factors

Sufferers of fibromyalgia report a number of situations or activities which trigger a flare-up of the condition and serve to aggravate their symptoms. In some cases these might be physical triggers, whilst in others they could be emotional or environmental. Being able to recognise your own triggers allows you to make changes to your lifestyle in order to avoid as many of them as possible, and keeping a diary of your symptoms and what was happening on each day can be an extremely useful way to pin them down.

Towards the end of 2005, an internet survey was carried out to find out, amongst other things, what were the key factors to aggravate the symptoms of fibromyalgia. A total of 2,569 fibromyalgia sufferers responded to the survey and, although the majority of these individuals were located in the United States, responses were also received from Canada, the United Kingdom, Ireland, Australia, New Zealand, Mexico, Germany, Holland, Bermuda, France, Israel and Hungary. While respondents were allowed to list as many aggravating factors as they wished, the four most common ones to be identified were mental stressors, weather changes, sleeping problems and strenuous activity. In this chapter, we will take a look at each of these, along with a number of others which have frequently been reported by fibromyalgia patients.

Stress

Although stress is an essential component in our lives in terms of allowing us to react appropriately in situations which might be dangerous to us, or in order to motivate us to get things done, when stress levels get too high they become unhealthy. As stress is one of the primary factors known to aggravate the symptoms of fibromyalgia (83% of the respondents to the above-mentioned survey quoted emotional distress as the main aggravating factor), it is important that sufferers are aware of their stress levels and that they do everything possible to keep them within healthy limits.

As anyone will understand who has suffered from the effects of stress, one of the things that we do quite unconsciously is to tense our muscles. Even for non-sufferers of fibromyalgia this can cause pain, soreness and headaches, but for those who do have the condition it can spark off episodes when the pain becomes very much more severe and is present for longer periods of time. While some believe that this muscle tension is the main reason why stress acts as an aggravating factor, others think that fibromyalgia sufferers react badly to the release of hormones which are produced during times of stress, and that these hormones interfere with the way in which pain is perceived by the body.

Of course, everyone has different perceptions of what constitutes a stressful situation, but for those who suffer from fibromyalgia it is particularly important that they be aware of their own stress triggers. These may not always be major events or situations such as tremendous emotional upheaval or unmanageable workloads, but could even be minor things such as excessive or constant noise. Once the causes of stress have been identified, sufferers then need to try and limit them, such as by reducing workloads, taking regular breaks or physically removing themselves from loud or vexatious situations. Listening to relaxing music or special relaxation tapes can be highly beneficial for many, as can practising meditation or yoga.

Unfortunately for sufferers of fibromyalgia, much of the stress that they experience is directly related to being diagnosed with the condition or the underlying fear that they may in fact be suffering from something far more serious. Where this is the case, education and communication are the keys to accepting the condition and reducing stress levels, something which is particularly important because prolonged exposure to stress can, of course, eventually lead into depression and anxiety, themselves common characteristics of the condition. Taking action early to minimise the effects of stress can go a long way towards ensuring that depression and anxiety are not allowed to take hold.

Weather Changes

Changes in weather conditions was the second most significant factor to be cited as an aggravator of fibromyalgia symptoms, with 80% of respondents stating that this causes headaches, muscle pain, morning stiffness and depression to worsen.

Cold, damp or humid weather conditions are all known to have huge potential to trigger or aggravate fibromyalgia symptoms, and some even find that they are particularly sensitive to changes in barometric pressure. Cold or draughty environments can also be a problem, so many sufferers find it beneficial to wrap up warmly in colder weather and to avoid sitting in corners or close to doors or windows where draughts are most likely to enter. In extreme cases, some have even moved to foreign shores where warm, dry climates have helped immensely to ease their symptoms.

Sleeping Problems

Sleeping problems such as insomnia and sleep apnea and the continual waking due to restless leg syndrome (RLS), periodic limb movement disorder (PLMD), muscle cramps, spasms and night sweats, can all have a huge impact, not only on the levels of pain that fibromyalgia sufferers experience during the day and the night, but also on the extent of morning stiffness and, of course, levels of fatigue.

Strenuous Activity

Revising expectations and understanding their own limitations are two things which fibromyalgia sufferers frequently have difficulty with. Having been perfectly able to undertake certain tasks or activities in the past, they expect to be able to continue with them in just the same way. The reality is, however, that what previously felt like normal levels of exercise and physical activity are likely to induce extreme fatigue, as well as increasing the severity of muscle pain. Anything which involves the repetitive use of muscles or the prolonged tensing of muscles requires particular caution, and many sufferers find it helpful to time their activities and change what they are doing regularly, so as not to put too much strain on a single part of the body.

By being vigilant and recording bouts of pain in a diary or journal, sufferers can get a clearer picture of what types of activities act as a trigger and so can change their lifestyles accordingly. In addition, they should avoid over-committing themselves to avoid rushing around and overdoing things.

Inactivity

Learning to get the balance right is vital in terms of minimising the symptoms of fibromyalgia and avoiding painful flare-ups, because inactivity, as well as overexertion, is a common aggravating factor.

Owing to the fact that fibromyalgia not only causes immense pain, but also muscle stiffness and restricted movement, many fibromyalgia sufferers are tempted to give up on exercise altogether. This, however, can actually aggravate the symptoms, and so what is called for are short, regular and gentle periods of exercise. Apart from anything else, without these, patients can often gain weight, something which again only causes deterioration in the condition.

Not only is regular exercise recommended to counteract periods of inactivity, but it is also important for individuals with fibromyalgia to take regular breaks from activities which might otherwise see them immobile for prolonged periods of time. Sitting at a computer for hours on end, for example, can cause back muscles to tense and can trigger a flare-up of symptoms, as can long car or train journeys or flights. Wherever possible, take a break roughly every 20 minutes and switch to doing something different or just walk around and do some gentle stretching exercises to prevent muscles from becoming stiff and sore.

Poor Posture

When we suffer pain as a result of injury or illness, the natural tendency is to change the way that we walk, sit or hold ourselves generally, in order to try and alleviate the discomfort. Compensating for the pain in these ways, however, can throw the entire body out of alignment, with the result that muscle pain and fatigue are actually increased.

For fibromyalgia sufferers, who are frequently in severe pain, it is important that posture is not dismissed as an issue as it can have an extremely detrimental effect in terms of aggravating pain symptoms. With a combination of pain management and special exercises to improve posture, the temptation to sit or move in unnatural ways can largely be removed.

Smoking

Alongside all the other widely publicised and harmful effects of inhaling smoke, nicotine and a huge number of chemicals into the body, smoking has the effect of reducing the amount of oxygen circulating in the bloodstream. Essentially, this not only starves the muscles, but also interferes with their ability to repair themselves efficiently, so adding to the amount of pain which is experienced by fibromyalgia sufferers. Some also report that nicotine in the body may also be linked to muscle contractions which, if experienced during the night, can cause sleeplessness and further aggravate the symptoms of the condition.

While some find that stopping smoking can be difficult, the resulting improvement in the levels of pain and the severity of other symptoms can be more than enough in terms of pay-off.

Hormonal Fluctuations

As we have already mentioned, it is possible that stress and other factors can bring about hormonal fluctuations which aggravate fibromyalgia symptoms. For women, however, it is often those which are associated with the premenstrual and menopausal states, as well as with pregnancy, which can give rise to a worsening of the symptoms of the condition.

Other Factors

The range of factors which can aggravate the symptoms of fibromyalgia is easily as wide, if not wider, than the range of symptoms itself, and of course everyone will have their own unique triggers. Although the factors that we have looked at here are the main ones to be reported by sufferers, it is important to pay attention to your own reactions to different environments, substances and situations so that you can determine what to avoid. Infections, allergies, physical injuries, time zone changes, chemical exposures, sexual intercourse and the side effects of medication are all additional factors which were highlighted by respondents to the 2005 internet survey as causing flare-ups, so try to pinpoint precisely what sets off your symptoms and then make adjustments to your lifestyle so that these can best be avoided.

9

The Top 7 Fibromyalgia Myths

With such a wide variety of symptoms, no known cause, no single definitive test and so many other similar conditions, in many ways it is not at all surprising that numerous myths have sprung up concerning fibromyalgia. To round off Part I of this book, therefore, let us just take a quick look at some of the most common ones in an attempt to separate fact from fiction.

Myth No 1 – It's All In Your Head
Being told that their problem is a psychological one is probably one of the most frustrating things for fibromyalgia sufferers who feel their pain to be not only real but severe. Although there is still much to be learned about the condition, extensive psychological tests have shown that its origins do not lie in the mind, and indeed the diagnosis of the condition is based on meeting very specific criteria, including the existence of a number of tender points at particular locations around the body.

Myth No 2 – I Can't See It, So It Doesn't Exist
Although not such a common response from doctors these days, this can sometimes be the reaction of family, friends, bosses and colleagues, who can be quick to assume that sufferers are 'putting on' their symptoms to avoid work or responsibilities around the home. What makes this myth all the more difficult to dispel is the fact that symptoms often come and go and vary considerably in their intensity from hour to hour and day to day. Although it can be hard to convince others that you are incapable of tackling certain tasks today when you felt fine yesterday, education and open and honest communication are key to securing their understanding and support.

Myth No 3 – Fibromyalgia Is a Middle-Aged Woman's Disease

Although the vast majority of fibromyalgia sufferers are women, between 10% and 20% of sufferers are men. In addition, whilst it typically strikes those between the ages of 20 and 55, children, adolescents and the elderly can all fall prey to the condition.

Myth No 4 – Fibromyalgia Is a Form of Arthritis

Arthritis is a condition which attacks the joints of the body, whereas fibromyalgia affects the muscles, tendons and ligaments.

Myth No 5 – Fibromyalgia Causes Serious Damage to the Body

In fact, fibromyalgia has been shown to cause no detectable physiological damage to the body at all, which is one of the reasons why it is so hard to diagnose. The symptoms of the condition do, however, tend to get progressively worse if no action is taken to limit its effects, and this in itself can lead to an overall deterioration in an individual's quality of life as muscles become weakened through lack of activity and use.

Myth No 6 – Fibromyalgia Is a Fatal Condition

There is no evidence whatsoever to suggest that fibromyalgia in any way shortens an individual's normal life expectancy.

Myth No 7 – As There Is No Cure for Fibromyalgia, There Is No Point in Seeing a Doctor

While it is true that there is currently no cure for fibromyalgia, there is much that can be done to limit the severity of the symptoms and make life more bearable. Doctors and pain specialists can not only investigate the use of a variety of traditional medications, but in addition they can suggest a range of alternative treatments and lifestyle changes which may well bring about immense benefit. You should always seek the advice of your doctor anyway, because diagnosis is difficult and the symptoms that you are experiencing may relate to completely separate illnesses which require entirely different courses of treatment.

Part Two

Myofascial Pain Syndrome –
Understanding the Basics

10

What Is Myofascial Pain Syndrome?

Although some sources quote myofascial pain as an alternative name for fibromyalgia, this is in fact incorrect. While the two disorders are in some ways similar, are often known to co-exist and may even be related, they do have different symptoms and require different methods of diagnosis and treatment.

Most people experience muscle pain at some points in their lives, but usually it clears up of its own accord within a matter of days. Those who suffer from myofascial pain syndrome (MPS), however, have muscle pain which is persistent or gets worse over time. Like fibromyalgia, MPS is a chronic, non-fatal, non-inflammatory condition, but in this case it is believed to affect the fascia or connective tissues which cover the muscles. With no known cause or cure and great difficulties being experienced in diagnosing the condition, it is another illness which some doctors have difficulty in accepting as being a 'real' disorder.

Although often equally severe, myofascial pain differs from the widespread pain which is associated with fibromyalgia. In MPS, the pain centres around what are known as 'trigger points', which are quite distinct from the 'tender points' found in fibromyalgia sufferers. Trigger points can be felt as nodules or rope-like bands under the skin and they can either be active or latent, causing either referred or localised pain.

When they are active, touching or pressing trigger points will cause referred pain (pain which is felt in a different area of the body) and possibly referred tenderness. In this state, they tend to cause continual pain, a reduction in muscle elasticity and muscle weakness.

Active trigger points can sometimes give rise to secondary or satellite trigger points which develop within the zone of referred pain. In this way, a localised pain pattern can spread to other and larger areas of the body.

When trigger points are latent, any pressure which is applied to them will normally only cause tenderness in that particular spot, but the pain will not be referred. Although the pain associated with latent trigger points tends to be less severe and less constant, they can cause stiffness and restricted range of motion. Latent trigger points do not necessarily remain latent, but can become active for a number of reasons which are thought to include muscle tension, psychological stress and physical factors such as poor posture.

Myofascial pain can affect any of the skeletal muscles in the body, but typically it causes regional pain in the neck, shoulders, lower back, pelvis, arms and legs. In addition, it is a common cause of headaches, as well as jaw and facial pain, something which has not only led to much research being carried out by the medical profession, but also by those in the field of dentistry. As distinct from the overall pain experienced by fibromyalgia sufferers, many report that myofascial pain is only felt in limited areas of the body, such as only down one side or in the neck and shoulder area. Having said this, however, the pain is not necessarily static and it can change location from one part of the body to another from day to day, as well as triggering different types of pain sensations.

In common with fibromyalgia, MPS is still somewhat of a mystery to scientists and those in the medical fields, but there is much research underway to uncover its origins and, hopefully, to develop a cure. In the meantime, pain management through a variety of medications and treatments, as well as certain lifestyle changes, have been shown to be highly effective in reducing the symptoms so that the impact on the quality of sufferers' lives is not so severely affected.

11

How Common Is Myofascial Pain Syndrome and Who Does It Affect?

Although statistics on the incidence and prevalence of MPS do vary, it is generally considered to be a very common illness. In fact, it is believed that almost everyone will develop at least one trigger point in their body at some point during their life, although in most cases the symptoms do not become severe enough to have any great impact on normal daily life.

Like fibromyalgia, MPS can affect the young and the elderly alike, as well as both sexes, and is most commonly reported by those who are in their twenties up to around the age of 50. There is also a similarity in that both conditions appear to see a peak in middle age, with some sources noting that it appears to be more common amongst those middle-aged people who are less active.

While many of the reported findings in relation to gender suscept-ibility state that there is an equal prevalence of myofascial pain in men and women, others incline towards a slightly higher ratio in females, although this does not seem to be nearly as pronounced as in fibro-myalgia.

12

Myofascial Pain Syndrome – The Symptoms

Myofascial pain syndrome, even though it is not an inflammatory or degenerative condition, can still present the sufferer with a range of distressing symptoms, the main one of which is pain which can range from being mildly uncomfortable to severe and incapacitating, and which can change location within the body. Typically the pain is described as being dull and non-pulsating, or like an ache which is felt deep inside the muscle. Throbbing or stabbing pains and burning sensations similar to those experienced with fibromyalgia have, however, also been reported.

As we have described, depending upon whether trigger points are latent or active, the pain which is experienced could be either local to the area of the trigger point itself or referred from a trigger point elsewhere in the body, and it could be either persistent or spasmodic. Whichever is the case though, it can generally, although not always, be felt both when the sufferer is at rest and active.

In addition to the pain which is characteristic of the condition, trigger points can also create a number of other symptoms, some of which may appear to be unrelated, such as:

- ▓ Stiffness in the muscle itself or in a joint close to the affected muscle
- ▓ An area of tension in the muscle which feels like a knot and may be very sensitive to the touch
- ▓ Numbness which is felt particularly in the extremities
- ▓ Muscle twitches when the trigger points are touched
- ▓ Restricted movement of the joints which is often experienced in the jaw

- Muscle weakness which can be so severe as to cause sufferers to drop things
- Trembling in the arm or leg, particularly as the limb is about to be used
- Clicking or popping of the joints
- Tension-type headaches
- Migraines
- Problems with balance
- Tinnitus and ear pain
- Changes in skin temperature
- Sweating
- Goose bumps
- Discharge of tears
- Salivation
- Memory dysfunction
- Double or blurred vision
- Nausea, dizziness and sweating

In many cases, these symptoms, along with the pain, will also lead to sleep disturbances as the sufferer struggles to find a comfortable sleeping position or hits a trigger point when they move during the night, so causing them to wake prematurely. Long-term muscle weakness is also another complication which can arise from the condition, because the pain discourages the use of the affected muscle which then begins to lose its strength. In fact, it is not uncommon for patients with MPS to develop all kinds of reflexes and protective habits to avoid activating the pain.

Depression and/or anxiety are not uncommon in sufferers of the condition either, perhaps as a direct result of being in constant and chronic pain. Anxiety in particular can be the cause of much distress as it has the potential to start off a vicious cycle. The tensing of muscles which is characteristic of anxiety sufferers is thought to contribute to the development of trigger points, thus causing more pain and more anxiety.

Whether MPS merely co-exists with or actually develops into fibromyalgia is not known, but a great many patients are found to suffer from both conditions, which of course only adds to their distress. Being very similar to one another, as well as to a range of other illnesses, physicians often find it difficult to make an accurate diagnosis and so patients can often go for long periods of time in a great deal of pain and without appropriate treatment. In addition, the pain which is experienced with MPS can contribute to and aggravate that associated with fibromyalgia, causing even greater impairment to the individual's quality of life.

13

What Causes Myofascial Pain?

The cause of MPS, like the cause of fibromyalgia, has led to much speculation over the years and, once again, the jury is still out. Research is still ongoing, however, and scientists in the fields of medicine and dentistry are attempting to get to the bottom of an illness which costs governments and businesses vast sums of money in terms of health care, lost productivity and absence from work. In this chapter, we are going to look at some of the theories that they have been working on.

Accidents and Injuries

One of the most common theories as to the cause of MPS is that it arises in the wake of accidents and injuries. Motor vehicle accidents, and particularly those involving whiplash type injuries, and falls are both thought to be directly responsible for the onset of the condition. The rationale behind this hypothesis is that accidents such as these can cause the muscles to stretch and then contract suddenly and violently, the effect of which is that the muscle fibres become tangled, shortened and stuck so that they do not release in the way that they should, even when the muscle is relaxed. The sensitive areas of tight muscle fibres which are created are the trigger points, with their characteristic tight, hard bands under the surface of the skin, and these cause strain and pain throughout the muscle, particularly if it is stretched suddenly again. The accident victim then begins to avoid the stretching motion so as not to experience the pain, which encourages the muscle to stay shortened, the trigger point to remain sensitive and the problem to continue.

Abnormal Muscle Stress

The theory concerning the overuse of muscles follows much the same line of thinking as that for accidents and injuries and, where it relates to the overuse of a particular muscle, the result is what we know as repetitive strain injury. Repetitive strain injuries are not only believed to cause the formation of new trigger points, but also to activate latent ones. Although in some cases such injuries can lead to inflammation of the overused tissues, this is not always the case and the pain actually comes from the trigger points created when the muscles, ligaments and fascia have become sore and irritated due to overuse.

Abnormal muscle stress, however, is not always self-inflicted through repetitive activities. In some cases, skeletal abnormalities such as having legs of different lengths or feet or toes of different sizes can cause certain muscles to receive harsher treatment than others and lead to the development of new trigger points and the resulting myofascial pain.

Poor Posture

Poor posture and/or sitting still for prolonged periods of time, is also thought to be the cause of the formation of trigger points. People whose jobs involve sitting at a computer and using a keyboard for lengthy periods, for example, can often impose undue stress on their shoulders, neck, upper arms and forearms. As the pain starts to worsen, they then try to compensate by adopting unnatural postures or completely immobilising the painful area, which adds to the soreness and discomfort as the muscle effectively gets stuck. As we said earlier, the onset of MPS seems to affect greater numbers of middle-aged people who are particularly inactive, and this theory certainly might help to explain why.

Stress and Anxiety

When we carry around feelings of stress and anxiety, commonly our muscles feel tense and locked. When the tension is chronic or when we feel this way for months or even years on end, this too is thought to cause the formation of painful trigger points, particularly around the neck and shoulder areas.

In some cases, the stress might arise directly as a result of the pain caused by an already activated trigger point. When we tense the affected muscle, however, this starts off a vicious cycle as the tension causes more pain, which in turn leads to more stress and so on.

Depression

While depression has been shown not to be a cause of fibromyalgia, there is a school of thought which links the depression frequently experienced by sufferers of the condition with MPS. In cases where fibromyalgia patients become depressed because of the constant pain and the severe restrictions imposed by the illness on their lifestyles, the level of serotonin in their brains drops. As serotonin is a neurotransmitter which is responsible for regulating not only mood but also pain, and as some believe that MPS is caused by the body's inability to interpret pain correctly, a drop in levels could actually be a cause of the condition, rather than an effect.

Nutritional Deficiencies

Nutritional deficiencies are another possible cause of MPS, and indeed as many as one in four patients suffering from a range of chronic pain ailments has been found to be deficient in vitamin D in particular. Vitamin D helps to protect against muscle weakness, as well as regulating the balance and absorption of calcium and phosphate in the body. While a deficiency may not on its own be responsible for causing MPS, many believe that it is responsible for an increase in the severity of chronic pain however. Just because blood tests show vitamin D levels to be within the normal range though, does not necessarily mean that you do not have MPS.

Low levels of iron, calcium, potassium, vitamin C and various of the B vitamins may also have a part to play in either causing or helping to alleviate the symptoms of MPS. Magnesium deficiency, which is believed to be responsible for chronic fatigue, chronic pain, insomnia, depression, cognitive dysfunction, anxiety and depression, IBS and digestive dysfunction, tremors and a whole range of other problems, could also prove to be key, as this element plays a vital role in assisting the transmission of nerve and muscle impulses.

Whether nutritional deficiencies actually cause MPS or other chronic pain illnesses is not at all clear, but adjustments to diet and the use of supplements certainly seem to have beneficial effects in terms of reducing pain levels for many people. As what we take into our bodies can not only determine how well our muscles, organs and so on heal themselves, but may also contribute to damage to the nervous system, particularly because of the toxins and chemicals which are introduced into our food, ensuring that we have a healthy diet is always a wise and sensible precaution.

Other Infections and Illnesses

Chronic infections, hypothyroidism, hypoglycaemia (abnormally low blood sugar level), conditions which cause damage to the nerve roots which connect the spine to the rest of the nervous system and diseases of the internal organs have also been implicated as causes for MPS, although no conclusive evidence exists as to how or why.

Connective tissue disease, which produces damage to the collagen and elastin which are the two main components of connective tissues, has also been cited as a possible cause. Elastin is what helps ligaments and muscles to stretch and then return to their original length.

The muscle contractions which occur around tender points in fibromyalgia patients may eventually cause trigger points to develop and so lead to MPS. In addition, restricting movement or adopting an unhealthy posture to limit fibromyalgia pain can also cause them to form.

Sleep Deprivation

As with fibromyalgia, sleep disorders and sleep deprivation can be a side effect of MPS and can aggravate both conditions. In MPS, both the persistent pain and the pressure on trigger points as the sufferer moves around in the night can cause severe restlessness, and the lack of sleep itself is believed to increase the sensation of pain.

Some believe, however, that both illnesses can actually stem from sleep deprivation, although the reasoning behind this theory does vary. The underlying causes of sleep disorders may in some way contribute to the onset of the condition, or it may simply be that the stress and anxiety of not being able to sleep may be the cause.

Oral Habits

The reason why the dental profession has put so much time and effort into the research of MPS is because the condition causes huge numbers of sufferers to experience pain in the face and the jaw and the condition may well be related to temporomandibular joint disorder (TMJD).

TMJD, the term used to describe acute or chronic inflammation of what is essentially the jaw joint, causes many of the same symptoms as MPS, including:

- A dull, aching pain in the face
- Jaw pain or tenderness in the jaw
- Restricted ability to open and close the mouth
- Neck and shoulder pain
- Headaches
- Tinnitus

Repetitive and unconscious movements of the jaw, a misaligned 'bite' or the lack of an overbite, jaw thrusting, persistent gum chewing or nail biting and trauma, as well as degenerative joint disease, can all play a part in TMJD, but could also be responsible for the formation of trigger points. As satellite trigger points can develop within the area of referred pain from active trigger points, it is possible that the pain could begin from the jaw and spread to other areas of the body to cause more widespread myofascial pain.

14

Diagnosing Myofascial Pain Syndrome

Because MPS is currently so poorly understood, diagnosis can often be difficult and sufferers can frequently experience long periods when they are not receiving appropriate treatment or are left feeling unsure as to how to manage the condition. As with fibromyalgia, there is no definitive laboratory test or X-ray to help make or confirm a diagnosis, although certain blood tests can be used to rule out other illnesses or to point to such things as nutritional deficiencies, the correction of which may help to alleviate chronic pain symptoms.

Diagnosis of MPS can be carried out quite effectively through the examination of a patient's medical history and clinical examination. As many physicians lack adequate training in relation to the condition, and some do not even accept it as a genuine disorder, it can sometimes be rather hit and miss however. In some cases, sufferers can find themselves moving from specialist to specialist before they receive an accurate diagnosis.

Medical History

Before doing anything else, your doctor should take the time to enquire about your general medical history, as well as to ask you some questions which are directly related to your current symptoms. The kind of areas that he or she is likely to cover might include:

- The symptoms that you are experiencing
- The length of time that you have been experiencing them
- Whether the pain and other symptoms are persistent or spasmodic
- The areas of the body where you feel the most severe pain

- Whether anything seems to make the symptoms either better or worse
- Whether the symptoms are worse at any particular time of the day, such as in the mornings
- Whether you have recently sustained any injuries
- Whether you perform any repetitive activities either at work, at home or during the course of your hobbies
- Whether the pain causes you to limit your activities

Before approaching a doctor, it can often be useful to consider these questions in advance and to keep a record or a diary of your symptoms. In this way, you will be able to provide much more accurate responses relating to a longer period of time, rather than just your most recent impressions.

Clinical Examination

Having investigated the range of symptoms that you are experiencing and the background to them, your physician is then likely to carry out a clinical examination. Although there are specific things that he or she will do and be looking for in relation to MPS, other types of test may also be carried out during the examination to rule out the possibility of other conditions.

The most reliable way to diagnose MPS is through the location and manual manipulation of trigger points. Because these tend to appear in fairly characteristic locations (over 70% of them correspond with the acupuncture points which are used to treat pain), locating them should not normally present too much of a problem and sensitive areas should show themselves fairly readily when gentle and consistent pressure is applied. The doctor will check your reactions as he or she explores the various points on your body, and you may experience a jolt of pain which causes you to flinch when sensitive areas are found. He or she may use a pressure algometer (which measures the amount of pressure that is being applied) in order to ensure that the pressure applied is consistent across all trigger points.

Having located the trigger points, the doctor will then palpate or manipulate them in order to detect the presence of nodules under the surface of the skin and knots or rope-like areas of muscle, and he or she may use three different techniques to achieve this. Direct finger pressure and flat palpation will help to examine the surface of the muscle, while pincer palpation will allow evaluation of the deeper layers. Where referred pain is detected, it may take between two and five seconds before the pain is felt, but the distinct pattern of pain will be the same each time the palpation is repeated. Manipulation of the trigger points may in addition cause muscle twitches, and localised sweating, temperature changes and other sensory reactions may also be experienced. This part of the examination may also be carried out by using needle penetration rather than manual palpation.

In some cases, physicians have been known to use other types of complementary tests to help with their diagnosis, including ultrasound, electromyography (which detects the electrical activity in the muscles) and thermography (to detect the levels of heat produced in specific parts of the body), but many question whether these do in fact provide any additional value above and beyond the more traditional clinical examination.

~

Clearly, in the course of diagnosing MPS, it is essential that doctors rule out other possible causes of your symptoms, as well as an underlying condition which might be causing it, and this may mean that you will have to undergo other types of test or examination. Because muscle pain can be caused by many different things, however, it is important that these tests are done so that an accurate diagnosis can be made as quickly as possible and effective treatment can commence.

15

Triggers and Aggravating Factors

Of course, the very nature of the trigger points associated with MPS means that all it takes to spark off pain is for pressure to be applied in just the wrong place. This can happen, for example, when adjusting position in bed at night or when a trigger point is knocked or bumped accidentally.

In addition, however, there is a range of things which can aggravate the condition and which can turn the less painful latent trigger points into active ones, causing persistent and referred pain. As you will see, however, many of the aggravating factors are, in fact, also potential causes of the condition.

Overuse of Muscles

Overloading the muscles, such as by lifting something which is too heavy or indulging in any type of vigorous physical activity or exercise can bring on or exacerbate the symptoms of MPS. Active stretching, such as that required to reach an item on a high shelf, can also trigger bouts of pain.

Direct Trauma

Direct trauma, such as through a fall or an accident can not only knock existing active trigger points and cause pain, but also lead to the formation of additional ones. Compensatory movements or immobilising parts of the body to take account of any bumps and bruises which might be sustained can also aggravate symptoms.

Prolonged Muscle Contraction

Long spells of immobility, and particularly those which involve too much time spent working at a single task such as typing or data entry, can cause the muscles to contract and become locked, so causing more intense pain. Anything which leads to prolonged muscle contraction, however, can have the same effect, including such activities as walking a long distance while carrying grocery bags.

Changes in Weather Conditions

As with fibromyalgia, changes in weather conditions can also aggravate myofascial pain. Sudden coldness and even sitting in draughts can cause the worsening of symptoms, and probably in part because cold tends to make us tense our muscles. Some people, however, also find that a damp environment, high humidity or extreme dryness will make their condition feel worse, although local warming of the trigger point has been known to help.

Viral Infections

There are several ways in which viral infections might lead to the aggravation of myofascial pain symptoms, even leaving aside any underlying physiological reasons. In many cases, the infections themselves can cause aches and pains in the body, which just add to the existing soreness and discomfort, but also the changes in body temperature and the inability to sleep well may contribute to activating trigger points.

Emotional Distress

Any kind of emotional distress or feelings of anxiety can cause tension in the muscles and so irritate trigger points.

∼

Although there is no known cure for MPS, there are many effective treatments that a good pain management specialist can help you with and we will look at a range of these in Part 4 of this book. Being able to identify and eliminate the aggravating factors and triggers which affect you personally, however, can do much to reduce the severity of the condition.

16

Myofascial Pain Syndrome and Fibromyalgia – The Terrible Twosome

In theory, myofascial pain should perhaps not present such enormous difficulties in terms of diagnosis as it actually does, but because less research has gone into this condition than is the case for fibromyalgia, and because doctors have, in some cases, received little or no training in it, it often represents an enormous challenge. Unless physicians are competent at recognising the signs of referred pain, as well as the characteristic nodules and taut bands of muscle associated with MPS, there is the potential for misdiagnosis.

As we have seen, illnesses such as chronic fatigue syndrome, Gulf War Syndrome and even hypothyroidism can sometimes be easily confused with fibromyalgia because they have extreme fatigue as one of their common symptoms. Although sufferers of MPS do frequently experience poor quality of sleep due to problems with persistent pain and because of the activation of trigger points during the night, the chronic fatigue which is experienced day and night by sufferers of the other conditions is not usually evident.

Confusion between MPS and fibromyalgia, however, is a different story. Some doctors are, in fact, fairly certain that the two conditions are related, while others think that MPS may even be responsible for triggering fibromyalgia.

Not only are the symptoms of the two illnesses in some ways similar, but what makes diagnosis all the harder is the fact that most of the tender point sites which are found in fibromyalgia are also trigger points in MPS. In addition, even though fibromyalgia involves widespread pain and MPS more localised and referred pain, over the course of time myofascial pain sufferers can develop satellite trigger points which cover larger and larger areas of the body, making the pain feel more widespread.

One of the greatest factors of all to get in the way of accurate diagnosis, however, is the fact that many people experience both conditions simultaneously. In fact, reports suggest that as many as 72% of the people who have fibromyalgia may also have trigger points associated with MPS. One study which was conducted at Selcuk University in Turkey found that just over 40% of a group of patients suffering from cervical MPS (which is specific to the neck area) also had fibromyalgia.

Because of the similarities, not only between MPS and fibromyalgia, but also between fibromyalgia and several other chronic illnesses, those who find themselves suffering from chronic pain are well advised to be highly vigilant in terms of their symptoms and to keep a record of them. Often when we approach a doctor for help, it is the most recent or troublesome symptoms which come to the forefront of our minds, rather than any kind of pattern in how they present themselves. Remember, the more information you can provide, and the more accurate that information, the quicker and more accurate the diagnosis is likely to be.

Part Three

Living with Fibromyalgia and Myofascial Pain Syndrome

17

Physical, Emotional and Psychological Impact

Fibromyalgia and MPS might not be fatal, but they are chronic conditions which can not only undermine physical health, but emotional and psychological well-being too. Despite being some of the most common illnesses in modern society, they are either not taken seriously or are little understood by many laypeople and physicians alike, a fact which in itself can make them much harder for sufferers to cope with.

Although in many ways the physical, emotional and psychological impacts are all interlinked, for the purposes of this chapter we are going to look at them separately.

Physical Limitations

Regardless of whether it happens suddenly or progressively, there are few of us who are not fully conscious of being able to do less than we used to. Even throughout the natural process of ageing we do not forget that years ago we could walk further, lift heavier weights and work for hours longer in the garden – although sometimes it would be a blessing if we could.

While in some cases fibromyalgia and MPS can be quite mild, perhaps mimicking the 'symptoms' of growing older, in others they can present severe physical limitations which make even routine daily tasks either extremely difficult or completely impossible. Reports suggest that in fact around half of fibromyalgia patients have trouble with routine daily activities or are unable to perform them at all, and approximately 30—40% have had to change jobs or stop working altogether.

Excruciating pain, debilitating fatigue, severe restrictions to movement and a whole host of other distressing symptoms can turn the things that were once taken for granted into what feel like insurmountable challenges. Simple household chores like tidying, hanging out washing or pushing a vacuum around can knock out what little wind is left in a sufferer's sails, and doing the weekly shopping might just as well be climbing Mount Everest for the effort that it takes. Pushing forward despite the pain and fatigue, even if that is possible, only leads to more severe problems, and so in many cases sufferers simply feel forced to give in. They do not generally do so, however, without first having faced many months or even years of frustration and considerable emotional distress.

Emotional Distress

The emotional distress that sufferers of fibromyalgia and MPS experience hits at oh so many different levels. Feeling lousy all or most of the time and being restricted in what they can do physically brings not only an immense sense of frustration but also huge amounts of guilt, as others are left to pick up their share of work and responsibilities. Partners, friends and family are sometimes forced to take a back seat as the limitations imposed by the illnesses make themselves felt, and sufferers can soon find that they are beating themselves up emotionally for not being a better husband or wife/friend/parent or whatever. If forced to give up work, they can berate themselves for loading up the pressure on their partners, not to mention feeling like a complete failure for not being able to contribute financially to the household.

What makes many of these things worse for sufferers of these particular conditions, however, is the fact that many laypeople and physicians alike think of them as nothing more than mythical disorders which are not to be taken seriously. There are no visible symptoms to confirm that there is actually something badly wrong; because so little is known or understood about fibromyalgia and MPS, sufferers are highly unlikely to elicit the same kind of sympathy and understanding that those of a disease such as rheumatoid arthritis are likely to receive.

Typically, people who have fibromyalgia or MPS live with a great deal of fear, at least in the early days and particularly before and for a while after diagnosis. Undergoing batteries of tests which all come back negative leaves them fearing the worst and that they might have some far more serious and possibly fatal condition. Even as they do begin to accept the illnesses for what they are, then comes the fear of what life will be like in the future.

The very pain which is experienced with fibromyalgia and MPS in itself provokes an emotional response. When it is very severe it can make us feel not only upset and tearful, but even angry. 'Why me?' we want to know.

Of course, one of the real problems of living constantly with high levels of pain is that it sets up a vicious circle. The physical pain causes an emotional reaction which, as many studies have shown, manifests itself in further physical symptoms which create more pain and so on. By seeking diagnosis early, and by following the advice of recognised specialists in the field of pain management and treatment, however, sufferers can better avoid this cycle and minimise the impact of these conditions on their daily lives.

Psychological Damage

As we have said, despite what may have been thought years ago, psychological factors are not the cause of fibromyalgia or MPS. They may, however, contribute to the illnesses in one of several ways, and particularly if it is the case that certain individuals have a predisposition to the conditions.

Trauma and high levels of stress, particularly if they are experienced over a long period of time, are known to change the ways in which our bodies function. Certain hormones and chemicals, for example, can be released into our systems in greater quantities, while other parts of our systems can be slowed down. This could have the effect of making certain people more susceptible to fibromyalgia and MPS or of triggering the onset of the conditions.

Some studies have shown that fibromyalgia is more prevalent in people who have suffered either emotional or physical abuse. This may indicate that chronic stress and trauma play a significant role in the development of the condition, perhaps as the result of long-term exposure to increased levels of stress hormones.

Depression and anxiety, however, can also develop as a direct result of the pain and other symptoms of the conditions, the fears associated with them, the lack of support from friends, families and doctors and the difficulties in coming to terms with what might be much altered lifestyles. In this case, they may have the effect of perpetuating the illnesses and making the symptoms feel worse.

Living with depression and anxiety on a day-to-day basis can feel just as incapacitating as the physical symptoms of fibromyalgia and MPS. The feelings of hopelessness and despair which are characteristic of depression can make getting out of bed in the mornings feel like a pointless exercise, and the fear, nervousness and worry which come with anxiety can turn even the most 'normal' situations and events into terrifying ordeals. Work, home life, relationships and hobbies can all suffer badly as a result, sending the sufferer into an ever deeper downward spiral.

Sadly, in some cases where the symptoms of fibromyalgia and MPS are left untreated and depression and anxiety are allowed to set in, individuals seek solace or 'solutions' through alcohol, drugs, the overuse of sleeping tablets or other forms of self-medication. Although these options might appear to offer some temporary relief, clearly they just add to the existing problems, and so it is important to turn to a specialist who is able to provide a holistic service and a range of treatments and therapies which can tackle the physical, emotional and psychological aspects of the conditions.

Around a third of fibromyalgia sufferers have been found to experience depression and/or anxiety, although it is not clear what proportion of these people may have been dealing with underlying psychological issues prior to their diagnosis. When considering treatment, therefore, it may be important not only to deal with any more recent depressive or anxious thoughts and feelings, but also to acknowledge any pre-existing psychological issues so that these too can be dealt with.

18

Impact on Relationships

Living with the physical, emotional and psychological effects of any chronic illness can have a profound impact on relationships, and not just those of the close and personal variety. Interactions with family members, friends, bosses and colleagues can all change dramatically and often not for the better.

As human beings, we all need relationships, but particularly with conditions such as fibromyalgia and MPS which few people understand, the temptation can be for sufferers to stop trying to communicate and to isolate themselves. In addition to the frustration of not being understood, they can also be fearful of the consequences of sharing underlying worries and concerns.

In this chapter we will look at the ways in which relationships are commonly affected by fibromyalgia and MPS, and then in Chapter 20 we will consider just what it is that those closest to you need to know and what they can do to help.

Family

Of all your relationships, it is typically those with your partner, children and close family members which are likely to be most affected by your illness. These are the people who will most often be at the sharp end of your irritability when the pain becomes difficult to handle and the ones who will find it hardest to revise their former expectations of you. They may even begin to feel as though they are living with someone completely different and may be left wondering 'What happened to the person that I used to know?' Frequently they will feel frustrated, helpless and angry, but it is important to remember that it is not you personally who is causing these feelings, but the illness.

With partners in particular, often what can happen is that the fibro-myalgia or MPS sufferer talks about the symptoms that he or she is experiencing, but fails to communicate the underlying fears and concerns. To the other party, this can come across as whingeing and complaining, and pretty soon they do not want to talk about the illness at all.

Talking to a partner about your fears concerning how the condition might affect your life in the future, however, can feel extremely difficult to do. What if he or she decides to up and leave? What if they decide to seek solace in another relationship, one which does not involve all the difficulties associated with chronic illness? Expressing your panic that you may even be dying from some other undiagnosed illness may make you feel as though you are being melo-dramatic, and so the emotions get bottled up and suppressed only to be vented in different and less constructive ways.

Because we are so close to our partners, it can be tempting to expect them to be mind readers, which of course they are not. Explaining rather than complaining, and asking for what you need, can go a long way to minimising the impact on your relationship with them. Even explaining that on some days you do not have the energy or the clarity of mind to explain can help to avoid possible miscommunica-tion.

With children, the issues can be quite different. Without any apparent rhyme or reason, children can often feel extreme guilt when a parent becomes sick. Somewhere in their little minds they imagine that it is something that they have done which has caused the illness, and when Mum or Dad is unable to play with them or attend to their needs in the same way as they did before, this simply compounds their fears. Feeling both guilty and pushed out, or even punished, they can sometimes react with attention-seeking behaviour which makes them much harder for the sick parent to handle. In other cases, they might become extremely withdrawn and fearful about what is going to happen in the future. As they watch their parent immobi-lised by pain and fatigue, they may not say it out loud, but inside they may be asking 'Is Mummy/Daddy going to die?'

Family members are a different story again, and their reactions might vary from extreme concern to telling you to pull yourself together. Often they will be quick to hand out advice, even though they know little or nothing about the condition that you are suffering from, and they may even take offence when that advice is not followed. This can be intensely frustrating for the sufferer, who may well find him or herself becoming snappy and irritable at their attempts to interfere. Usually, however, the reactions of family are born of nothing other than the very deepest concern for their loved one's well-being.

Friends

Friendships are precious, but in many cases they are not based on the unconditional type of love which is felt between partners and family members, which makes them all the more fragile. Having to turn down invitations to meet and spend time with friends can make them feel totally pushed out and rejected, especially if they understand little about your condition and how it affects your daily life.

Like partners and family, friends can also feel extremely helpless in the face of chronic illness, but because they are not so closely involved in the situation, this can cause them to withdraw. In addition, some can become fearful, almost as though the condition is contagious, which again might lead to them keeping their distance.

Physical Relationships

Aside from the other difficulties which can be experienced in close personal relationships, fibromyalgia and MPS can also have an effect on a couple's sex life, and this is an impact which is often overlooked. In some cases, the problems might be emotional ones which arise from a feeling of growing distance between the two partners, but in other cases it can be at the purely physical level.

Although not always the case, both men and women who suffer from fibromyalgia or MPS can sometimes experience a decrease in sex drive or even a complete loss of libido. Often this is associated with feeling stressed, depressed or anxious, but in women in particular it can have much to do with negative changes in self-image. The weight gain which frequently accompanies the illnesses can make them feel fat and unattractive, and the loss of muscle mass which is also sometimes experienced can leave them feeling flabby and untoned. In addition, lack of energy can lead some women to neglect their normal grooming and self-care regimes so that they might feel less inclined to put on make-up or dress up in a way which makes them feel attractive, which in turn can affect their self-esteem and sexual confidence. Even the loss of their normal sense of vibrancy can make them feel generally less appealing.

In a physical sense, chronic pain and fatigue can make any semblance of a normal sex life feel impossible. Aside from the persistent pain which can be felt in both conditions, in fibromyalgia, muscles can cramp and if this happens in the pelvic or lower back region, this can make intercourse uncomfortable at best and painful at worst. Once this has happened on several occasions, a woman may begin to associate sexual activity with negative feelings and so be inclined to avoid it. In MPS, any pressure on the trigger points can cause either localised or referred pain which can again make sexual intercourse painful. Where chronic fatigue is experienced, many sufferers do not have the physical energy to walk a hundred yards, let alone engage in sexual activity.

In some ways, fibromyalgia and MPS sufferers and their partners can find themselves in a Catch 22 situation. The medications which are prescribed to lift depression and anxiety or kill the pain might eliminate those particular barriers to sexual activity, but in many cases they can cause a decrease in sex drive or cause erectile dysfunction while they are being taken. On the other hand, while sex itself causes the release of hormones which have a positive effect on pain and depression, the loss of libido caused by the illness itself, as well as the pain and fatigue which are experienced can make it a highly unattractive proposition.

Of course, any effect on the physical relations between a couple will almost certainly impact on the emotional bond and levels of intimacy too, and so it is important that sufferers and their partners do not neglect this area of their lives. Here are a few tips to help you to minimise the impact of these two conditions on your physical and emotional bond.

■ Understand that there may be changes to your sex life and learn all you can about how these might affect you and your partner. In this way you will be better prepared to accept and deal with any problems which do arise.

■ Rather than pretending that the problem does not exist or just hoping that it will clear up of its own accord, talk to your partner about any fears, concerns or insecurities that either of you may have. This will allow you to maintain a close emotional and intellectual bond and will help to boost your sexual intimacy.

■ If sexual intercourse is uncomfortable or painful in one particular position, try experimenting with other positions.

■ Remember that physical relationships do not stop at sexual intercourse. Other directly sexual and non-sexual activities such as oral or manual sex and massages can do much to promote intimacy and relieve tension.

■ Knowing that the sufferer's self-esteem and feelings of desirability are likely to be affected, partners can offer their reassurance both inside and outside of the bedroom by treating his or her partner more often or offering compliments more frequently.

■ It is important not to make someone who is probably already struggling with their own feelings around sexuality feel pressurised, so partners can help by taking actions which are likely to make sex seem more appealing, rather than by being demanding or emotionally forceful.

■ Take advantage of the 'good days' or the good parts of the day when the symptoms are less severe, not just to hop into bed, but also to spend quality time together and put back some of the romance into your relationship.

■ People respond differently to medications, so if you suspect that the ones you are taking are causing problems with libido, do not be afraid to discuss this with your doctor. There may be other alternatives which have less of an effect .

Bosses and Colleagues

Trust in the workplace is important, but the trouble with illnesses which have no outward signs and which, despite being so common, many people have never heard of, is that sometimes they can leave bosses and colleagues wondering whether you might not be making up the symptoms you describe. Even if others have heard of fibromyalgia and MPS, because there is so much 'bad press' surrounding them, sufferers can still be thought of as malingerers or hypochondriacs and regarded with some suspicion.

Colleagues who have to pick up extra responsibility if a team member needs to take time off work on a fairly regular basis can also begin to feel bitter, and where special arrangements such as flexible working hours are permitted to 'work around' the illness, jealousy can be an issue too. Of course, if the individual were suffering from some better known illness which bosses and colleagues understood more about, there might be less of a problem, but the difficulty here is one of credibility.

19

Impact on Attitudes

Acceptance

You only have to talk to a sufferer of fibromyalgia or MPS to learn that one of the hardest things about being diagnosed with one of these conditions is accepting that they have it in the first place. Part of the reason for this lies in the fact that the conditions themselves are not widely accepted or understood. Patients are told that they have these weird illnesses that even those in the medical profession do not fully understand, but if doctors themselves find them hard to accept and cannot even explain how their patients came to contract them, how are the patients supposed to accept them?

Another huge reason why acceptance can often be difficult is, of course, because fibromyalgia and MPS are illnesses which have no known cure. At the same time as diagnosing these illnesses, doctors have to explain to their patients that they are going to have to live with these chronic conditions for the rest of their lives, news which many people find particularly difficult to come to terms with.

Particularly when the diagnosis of fibromyalgia and MPS has been a long, drawn-out affair during which the sufferer's mind has had ample time to run riot and imagine every horrible terminal illness in the book, often they expect to feel relieved to find out what is actually causing the problem. In reality though, when patients discover that they have a condition which is incurable and means having to cope with sometimes extreme levels of pain for the rest of their lives, it is denial that hits them, not relief. Instead of being able to accept what is happening, in some cases they just spend their lives wishing that someone would come along and wave a magic wand to make it all go away. In others, they put huge amounts of time and effort into chasing 'miracle cures' for their lifelong illness which do nothing more than relieve them of their cash and give them false hope. By allowing themselves to get caught up in denial, however, their physical symptoms often worsen as a result of the additional stress.

The degree to which sufferers of fibromyalgia and MPS are able to accept their conditions, though, will generally have a direct impact on how quickly and effectively they are able to manage their symptoms and so begin to live a relatively normal existence. To an extent, their acceptance and their handling of their situation will, of course, depend on their own make-up. Those who face it head-on with a positive frame of mind and a strong sense of determination often fare better and work harder to ensure that they have the necessary support systems in place and that their lives are arranged in such a way that the effects are minimised. Those who choose to live in denial, meanwhile, can become consumed with negativity and spend their lives fighting against their illness instead of learning to live with it.

Of course, much of an individual's reaction to a diagnosis will depend on his or her own personal circumstances, but incredibly there are those who manage to see their illness as the door to new opportunities. Those who are stuck in jobs that they hate or that they have been struggling for too long to manage, for example, can find themselves feeling relieved at the prospect of being able to explore new lines of work, perhaps in fields that they would never have considered in the past or only ever dreamed about. Optimists such as these look for the silver lining, and generally they find one.

For most people, however, there is almost bound to be some degree of difficulty in accepting a diagnosis of fibromyalgia and/or MPS, as there would be with accepting any other lifelong condition. Some have described the cycle as being the same as that which people go through in bereavement, with denial, anger, bargaining and depression all having to be faced before acceptance is finally reached. In learning to accept the illness itself, accept also that you are likely to go through each of these stages. The trick though, if there is one, is to feel the feelings and then move on to take control, and this is what we are going to look at next.

Staying Positive and Taking Control

Fibromyalgia and MPS really are two conditions which have the potential to take over your life, and that is a very scary prospect. Without making the effort to stay positive and maintain some sense of control, it is all too easy to allow your every conversation to be dominated by your illness and your every action dictated by it. If you let it, it will drag you down into despair and depression.

Constantly maintaining a positive attitude in the face of a lifelong illness is a huge challenge and there will inevitably be days where doing so simply feels impossible. The power of positive thought, however, has been proven time and time again in relation to a whole range of physical illnesses. Even in the case of what were diagnosed as terminal illnesses, patients have experienced long and unexpected periods of remission, lived well past their doctors' expectations or totally beaten their diseases. People who have been told that they would never walk again have turned their physicians' prognoses on their heads, and all through the power of positive thought and sheer grit and determination.

While, realistically speaking, maintaining a positive attitude in the face of fibromyalgia and MPS will not cure a sufferer of the condition, it does of course have the benefit of helping him or her to steer clear of depression and anxiety, two things which have the potential to make living with the conditions very much harder. Aside from this, however, studies have shown that those who do manage to think positively frequently experience a reduction in the severity of their symptoms.

As we mentioned in the previous section, passing through the five stages of denial, anger, bargaining, depression and, finally, acceptance, may be fairly inevitable, but there are things that those who are diagnosed with fibromyalgia and MPS can do to help them stay positive and take control. The first of these is something that you are doing right at this moment – arming yourself with knowledge – and the more you learn, the more in control and empowered you will feel. The second thing is to grieve if you feel the need to do so, but then move on. It is not silly or unacceptable to grieve for the loss of your former way of life, but there comes a point when the grieving has to stop and you have to get on with living.

The third thing that you can do to help yourself may take a little practice if you are not naturally inclined to think positively, but it can still be achieved with relatively little effort and just a little awareness. Change your focus so that instead of thinking about all the limitations that lie ahead in your life, you see them as being challenges to be overcome. There is a saying which goes, 'There are no problems, just situations', and getting into this mindset can really help to change your attitude for the positive. Instead of seeing problems as obstacles in life, focus on them as opportunities to do different things or to do things differently. Look past the immediate and the obvious and think creatively about how your life can be adjusted to make it more comfortable, manageable and pain-free. Try out the tips, suggestions, therapies and treatments that you will find in Part 4 of this book and explore what works for you. Rise to the challenge rather than letting your illness drag you down, and concentrate on the doable, not the impossible.

Also, do not let yourself become consumed by your illness and feelings of negativity, but focus instead on the positives in your life such as your family, friends or a special hobby or interest that you may have. The world may seem to be a pretty bleak place at times, but there are still good things in your life, so acknowledge them and take pleasure in them.

Learning to live your life one day at a time is another key way to take control of your illness. Maybe today is a bad day, but it is just one rough day amongst other good ones, and tomorrow may be very much better. If you spend your life anticipating another bad day, the chances are that that is precisely what you will get, so just accept today for what it is and see what tomorrow brings.

Laughter, as they say, is the best medicine, so try not to lose your sense of humour in the face of your illness. Hang out with friends who make you laugh, watch your favourite comedy programmes and movies and generally enjoy your life as much as you can, because it really is not all bad.

20

What Friends and Family Need to Know and How They Can Help

As much as fibromyalgia and MPS are difficult for the sufferers them-selves to deal with, they can also have a profound effect on family and friends. Although perhaps to a lesser degree, it is not uncommon for them to also go through the five stages of grief in the face of their loved one's illness. In many cases they too will want to deny what is happening and feel angry about the changes that the illness will inflict on their own lives and the lives with their partners, parents, friends or whomever. They will almost certainly feel sad and low because they miss the 'old you', but in most cases they will want to help and support you too.

Feeling helpless in the face of someone else's illness is a horrible experience, and it does not have to be a serious or chronic illness for this to be the case. Any mother will know the feelings associated with trying to calm a baby who is screaming with colic pains, or watching a child suffer the agony of a migraine. It is not just helplessness, but sorrow and pity and even guilt. Did I cause it? Should I be doing something different to alleviate it?

Of course a baby cannot explain or reassure when it sees its mother's helplessness, and nor can it tell its mother what would help. As a fibromyalgia or MPS sufferer, however, you can and you should, for everyone's sake. Remember, these people might be able to see your suffering on the outside, but they cannot feel what you feel on the inside, physically, emotionally or psychologically. They are not mind readers either and without good communication on your part, they will not know what to do to ease your plight.

Your partner, children, family members and friends are the closest people to you and it is important to put your trust in them and to reach out to them. Here are a few useful tips on how to do just that.

Keep it simple

Although it will benefit both you and your loved ones if they know something about your condition, there really is no need to go into lengthy, in-depth explanations which cover all the ins and outs. Keep information basic and relevant to you, otherwise you not only risk blinding them with science or confusing them with medical terminology, but also causing them to shut down and stop listening.

Of course, there are essentials that you will need to cover, such as the fact that it is not life-threatening but is incurable, what your symptoms are and the ways in which the illness impacts on your life. When you describe your symptoms, try to relate these to things that they will understand, such as the aches and pains associated with a really bad bout of flu or what it feels like the day after a tough workout at the gym, the frustration of forgetting the simplest things and not being able to think clearly and how it feels when you cannot sleep for night after night. I read somewhere that one sufferer explained fibromyalgia as feeling as though your whole body has a migraine, which for many people probably sums it up quite nicely. You might also want to provide your loved ones with a brief overview of how the condition can be managed or the courses of treatment that you are following or investigating.

Point them in the right direction if they want to learn more

After you have explained in the simplest terms, there may be family members, friends, colleagues or employers who wish to learn more about your condition. If this is the case, share any valuable information in the form of brochures or print relevant information from the internet for them to read. If they do not ask, then resist the temptation to foist it upon them, but if there is a genuine desire to learn more, then point them in the right direction.

Don't complain – explain

When you talk to your friends and family, try to explain in a calm, matter-of-fact way rather than whingeing and whining, because the latter do nothing to help you get your point across and can often have the effect of making others feel less sympathetic.

Don't expect others to read your mind

Your loved ones might be close to you but they cannot read your mind. It is up to you to ask for what you need, whether that be help with the housework, for them to take the children off your hands for a while or whatever.

Also, remember that they may not appreciate how your symptoms impact on your mood, so let them know that feeling tired, irritable, agitated and forgetful are all symptoms of the condition which you do your best to control, but …

Don't use your family and friends to vent your negative feelings

It is one thing to explain that you might sometimes run short of patience, but it is quite another to take your negative feelings out on those closest to you. You may be sick, but your illness affects everyone around you to at least some degree and if you want those people to be supportive of you, you must continue to treat them with love and respect. After all, it is not theirs or anyone else's fault that you have the illness and all they really want to do is help.

Encourage their feedback

Living with a chronic illness involves a team effort and good communication from all the parties involved. Let your family and friends know that they do not have to tread on eggshells and that you are open to receiving a reality check when necessary. If that reality check then comes, take it on board.

Let them know to include you

The very nature of fibromyalgia and MPS is such that there are bound to be times when you have to cancel arrangements or turn down invitations because you simply are not up to them. You do not have to be sick, however, to understand that if you cancel or refuse often enough, people will simply stop asking. Let your family and friends know that you will make every effort to continue your life as normal, that any refusal should not offend and that they should not exclude you from their plans. Living with these conditions can become very isolating, so be sure to get across that you value greatly the time spent with them and would hate to feel left out.

21

Finding a Doctor Who Understands

As we have mentioned at several points throughout this book, there are still those within the medical profession who either misunderstand fibromyalgia and MPS or who are just sceptical about its existence per se. Trying to deal with these kinds of practitioners is, quite simply, soul-destroying. You have these terrible symptoms, you know that they are real and not all in your imagination and the last thing you need is for the very person who is supposed to be helping you, to treat you like a crazy person or with condescension.

In some cases, even doctors who believe in the illnesses but have little experience in them are reluctant to treat them because doing so would involve a significant amount of research on their part, such as into options for medication, as well as arranging all the necessary referrals. Frequently, however, patients find themselves settling for a doctor who believes in their condition, even if he or she is not able to provide them with the best treatment.

Finding a doctor who not only understands your condition, but is adept at diagnosing it and treating it is, though, essential if you are to maintain any semblance of a normal life and keep your sanity into the bargain. It is imperative that the physician you choose is somebody who is sympathetic to your needs and will listen to you and work with you to find the very best possible course of treatment. He or she needs to understand not only the complexity of the conditions, but also their impact on the lives of sufferers. If you do not feel that your current practitioner is doing all he or she can to help you, then it would be wise to consider an alternative.

While having an understanding GP is, of course, always a bonus, the fact is that many do not have the specialist knowledge of fibromyalgia and MPS that is required to manage the conditions effectively. Even some specialist physicians such as rheumatologists will claim to be able to treat these illnesses, but frequently even they are not experts and have little experience of dealing with them. Pain management specialists such as those at the London Pain Clinic, on the other hand, not only have a considerable number of years' experience in fibromyalgia and MPS, but they can provide a service which ranges from initial assessment, through the development of an individual treatment plan to holistic treatment using a wide range of traditional, alternative and cutting edge techniques, including such things as the use of Botox.

As you have seen, the range of symptoms experienced by sufferers of fibromyalgia and MPS are wide and varied, which adds greatly to the complexities of treatment. Treating one symptom can quite easily lead to flare-ups in others, and so thorough knowledge and experience in the field is critical in finding the right balance to achieve maximum effect for each individual.

Communicating with Your Doctor

With conditions such as fibromyalgia and MPS, effective communication between doctor and patient is crucial. Symptoms come and go, move around and appear as if from nowhere. Because treatment involves a multidisciplinary approach, it is vital too that all aspects are properly understood by the patient if they are to receive the greatest benefit. Here, therefore, are a few tips to help guide you in your communications with your expert specialist.

■ Prepare for your appointment by being able to outline your reasons for being there and by taking with you notes on your medical history and a list of any medications that you are currently taking.

■ Think in advance about how you are going to describe your symptoms – the type of pain, the nature of the fatigue, the pattern of sleeplessness, the restrictions to your movement, etc.

■ When you ask your doctor questions, try to avoid those which would require only a yes or no answer. Phrase your questions instead so that you get a fuller explanation which leaves you in no doubt.

- When your doctor provides a response, listen carefully and do not interrupt. If there is anything that you are unsure about, ask him or her to clarify the necessary points.

- When you return for follow-up appointments, be prepared to discuss the positive and negative effects of the various elements of your treatment plan. If it helps to remind you, keep a record of any changes in your symptoms and take this along with you.

- Your treatment plan may change along the way as your doctor tries different and potentially more effective alternatives or as new techniques become available, so be aware that your treatment is not likely to remain static.

- Understand that, for your treatment to be most effective, two-way communication is required and that you are responsible for your role in your treatment by following your treatment plan as outlined by your doctor and feeding back to him or her accurately.

Part Four

Treatment Options for Fibromyalgia and Myofascial Pain Syndrome

22

Treatment Options

In fibromyalgia and MPS, what we have are two chronic pain disorders which frequently go hand in hand, can often have a devastating effect on people's lives, but are currently without known cause or cure. The good news, however, is that there is a great deal that can be done to manage the symptoms of both conditions, and the various options encompass everything from treatment using traditional medications and physical therapies, through to more alternative and cutting-edge treatments, exercise, stress management, cognitive behavioural therapy, diet and, of course, education.

A couple of things which are really important to remember about treatment for these conditions, however, are firstly that the goal is to relieve and not cure symptoms, and secondly that there is no single treatment or combination of treatments which works for every sufferer. Treatment plans need to be specifically tailored to each patient's needs and it is only by doctor and patient working closely together that the best choices can be made for each individual. To begin with at least, treatment plans will often involve an element of trial and error to find out what does and does not work, and of course each patient's expectation of treatment and idea of what is an acceptable improvement will vary. With different symptoms waxing and waning at different times, this close working relationship between doctor and patient is crucial in allowing the former to make adjustments to the treatment programme as necessary.

A comprehensive, multidisciplinary approach is often the most effective for both fibromyalgia and MPS and so the patient can often find him or herself dealing with a range of different specialists. Indeed, this is one of the reasons why finding a practice which takes a holistic approach to treating the conditions makes far more sense as the whole treatment programme is far more 'joined up'. It can also help to avoid patients being prescribed with cocktails of drugs which might react with one another and, of course, with a single physician to oversee each case, it is much easier to determine the right combination of treatments to gain maximum relief from symptoms.

For the remainder of this chapter, therefore, we are going to look at an overview of the treatment options available for each of the conditions, and then in the rest of Part Four we will consider these options, as well as treatment of certain specific symptoms in greater detail.

Treatment for Fibromyalgia

Because chronic pain and fatigue are normally the two most significant and bothersome symptoms of fibromyalgia, most traditional treatments are geared towards decreasing the levels of pain and improving the quality of sleep. Different doctors and fibromyalgia associations recommend different ranges of treatments to achieve these ends, with the American Pain Society Fibromyalgia Panel, for example, suggesting a combined approach to treatment which incorporates education, cognitive behavioural therapy, medication and exercise. While the first two elements are designed to teach patients how to cope with the condition, to change their attitudes towards it and their coping methods, the latter two focus on relieving symptoms and increasing mobility. In some cases physicians prefer to start with medication and then progress to other types of treatment, whilst in others, drugs are only used if other methods fail to improve symptoms.

Generally speaking, drugs such as aspirin and cortisone, which are often used to treat musculoskeletal pain, do little if anything to impact on fibromyalgia pain and so a variety of other pain relievers, sleep medications, anti-convulsants and muscle relaxants have typically been prescribed for the condition. Antidepressants are also commonly prescribed, although not specifically to treat depression, but rather because of their ability to alter the levels of certain chemicals which are used to carry pain messages to and from the brain.

Stretching and aerobic exercise are commonly accepted as being significantly beneficial for sufferers of fibromyalgia, not least because the restrictions in movement caused by pain and stiffness can frequently lead to patients becoming out of condition. Exercise can also help to ease muscle spasms by improving blood flow and encouraging healing. Physiotherapy techniques such as massage, meanwhile, are used to treat muscle stiffness or weakness.

'Talk therapies' such as cognitive behavioural therapy and psychotherapy are typically aimed at changing the way that sufferers think about and handle things, as well as dealing with underlying issues, thoughts and feelings which might contribute to the stress, anxiety or depression which are commonly associated with fibromyalgia.

The list of alternative and complementary therapies and treatments is a long one, but many sufferers report significant improvements in their symptoms as a result of these. Some of the most common ones to be recommended include acupuncture, acupressure, herbs, nutritional supplements, water therapy, myofascial release therapy, relaxation techniques, yoga, breathing exercises, aromatherapy, hypnosis, the application of heat or cold and osteopathic or chiropractic manipulation.

Treatment for Myofascial Pain Syndrome

As with fibromyalgia, the treatment for MPS also generally takes a combined approach, which might include the use of medications, physical therapies and trigger point injections, although again some alternative remedies and treatments have also been found by some to be highly effective.

The prescription and non-prescription medications in the form of non-steroidal anti-inflammatory drugs which are tried by MPS sufferers are typically not very effective at relieving the pain. Tricyclic antidepressants have been shown to work to better effect and have also aided more restful sleep.

Physical therapies such as stretching exercises and massage are also focused on relieving pain but, in addition, therapists can also help patients to identify and correct, for example, poor posture which might be contributing to the problem. Trigger point injections, on the other hand, can help to relieve the tension which sufferers experience in the muscle.

Gentle exercise can help patients to cope better with the pain, while relaxation techniques can stop the stress and tension which contribute to the build-up of pain. Herbs, supplements and a range of other complementary and alternative treatments and therapies, including acupuncture, have also proven to be very effective for some.

Another treatment which is more commonly used for MPS is what are referred to as myofascial release techniques. These concentrate on releasing restrictions in the muscle fascia and restoring elasticity and hydration.

23

Medications and Contraindications

As we have said, it is widely recognised by those with greater experience in fibromyalgia and MPS that a combination of treatments tends to be more effective at relieving symptoms than any one single course of action. In many cases, a comprehensive treatment plan may well include certain types of prescribed or over-the-counter medications as part of a multidisciplinary approach, but it has to be said that those physicians with limited knowledge of the condition quite often rely entirely on these drugs to treat the broad range of symptoms which are typically experienced. Of course, the great danger here is that patients can often begin to feel like walking medicine cabinets as they ingest increasing numbers of tablets which sometimes have side effects, can become addictive and also have the potential to react against one another. That is not to say that there is no benefit to using medication, but it is vital, however, that it be prescribed with care and as part of a broader treatment package.

The types of medications which are commonly used by practitioners to treat the symptoms of fibromyalgia and MPS include those to help manage pain, fatigue and sleeplessness, any associated psychological distress that the patient may be experiencing and to increase mobility, as well as other drugs to alleviate related medical problems such as migraine and irritable bowel syndrome. In this chapter, we are going to look at some of the main categories of medication which are typically prescribed by doctors in the treatment of fibromyalgia and MPS, including pain relievers (analgesics), anti-convulsants, antidepressants, muscle relaxants, psychotropic drugs and sleep medications, as well as at some of the contraindications or side effects which are commonly experienced. Following this, we will go on to consider a whole range of other non drug-related, complementary and alternative treatments and therapies which have proven to be highly effective in lessening the symptoms of the two conditions.

Pain Relievers

Although non-prescription pain relievers such as aspirin and paracetamol can be effective for a range of conditions in which inflammation is a factor, they tend not to provide much relief for sufferers of fibromyalgia and MPS because these, of course, do not cause any inflammation in the joints or muscles. Although over-the-counter drugs might appear to be fairly safe, taking non-steroidal anti-inflammatory drugs (NSAIDs) such as these in large quantities or over prolonged periods of time and in an attempt to relieve pain symptoms can increase the risk of stomach ulcers and internal bleeding.

Narcotic pain killers or opioids such as codeine (a derivative of opium), morphine, hydrocodone and oxycodone, on the other hand, may offer greater relief for those with moderate to severe pain, but carry the danger of the patient becoming physically dependent and suffering withdrawal symptoms when the drug is discontinued. Opioids work by interfering with the transmission of the pain signals to the brain, and also by altering the way in which the brain perceives pain.

The most common side effects experienced while taking opioids include drowsiness, nausea and vomiting, dry mouth, itching, constipation and depression. In addition, the drug can affect libido or increase complications related to erectile dysfunction. In cases where an allergic reaction is experienced, individuals can develop skin rashes and swelling of the skin. In higher doses, codeine also has the potential to depress the respiratory system and can be particularly dangerous for babies who are being breastfed, as the drug is passed to the baby through the mother's milk in what could be lethal amounts. Many doctors consider the use of opioids in general for fibromyalgia and MPS to be highly controversial.

Tramadol, which is produced under the brand name of Ultram®, is a manmade or synthetic pain killer which is commonly prescribed to treat moderate to moderately severe pain in fibromyalgia and MPS sufferers, as well as that associated with other chronic pain conditions. The drug works by binding to certain receptors in the brain which are important for transmitting pain sensations throughout the body. Its side effects may include nausea, drowsiness, constipation or diarrhoea and dizziness and, although it is considered to be less addictive than drugs such as codeine, it does still carry some risk of physical dependence.

Tramadol is not recommended for pregnant women, nursing mothers or those who also suffer from heart or kidney disease or recurrent or chronic breathing conditions, as well as those who are taking certain other medications. When combined with certain other drugs such as the anti-convulsants Tegretol, Equetro and Carbatrol, the effects of tramadol are reduced. If taken alongside selective serotonin reuptake inhibitors (SSRIs) such as Prozac®, Zoloft® and Paxil®, meanwhile, patients can experience severe side effects such as seizures or a condition known as serotonin syndrome which can be fatal. Tramadol should also not be used in combination with tricyclic antidepressants.

Anti-Convulsants

The term 'anti-convulsants' refers to a wide range of medications which are designed to prevent seizure activity in the brain. Although different types of anti-convulsant drugs use different mechanisms to achieve this, most work by blocking different chemical messengers or neurotransmitters and by binding to different receptors in the brain.

One of the most common anti-convulsant drugs to be used in the treatment of fibromyalgia and MPS is pregabalin, which is sold under the trade name of Lyrica®. Approved by the European Union in 2004 and by the US Food and Drug Administration (FDA) one year later, it is often prescribed for sufferers of epilepsy and generalised anxiety disorders, but has additionally proved to be effective in reducing pain symptoms and improving sleep quality in those with fibromyalgia and MPS. In fact, one study showed that 63% of patients experienced reduced levels of pain as a result of taking Lyrica®.

Although most people who take Lyrica® experience few, if any side effects, the main active ingredient, pregabalin, can sometimes cause mild to moderate dizziness or sleepiness and impair motor function, as well as affecting concentration. For pregnant women or breast-feeding mothers and those who suffer from allergies, a history of drug abuse, eye disease such as glaucoma and kidney and heart disease, it is important that these are discussed with your doctor before taking this medication. Children and older adults and those who are scheduled for surgery of any kind should also be carefully assessed and monitored before pregabalin is prescribed.

Antidepressants

A range of antidepressants may be prescribed for sufferers of both fibromyalgia and MPS, not because either of these conditions are psychological illnesses, but because they address the deficiency of the neurotransmitter serotonin which is frequently found in patients with these conditions. Administered in much lower doses than would be prescribed for the treatment of depression, these drugs have been shown not only to help control the pain of fibromyalgia and MPS, but also to promote more restful sleep. In cases where patients are also suffering from depression, however, higher dosages may be used.

The three main types of antidepressants which are prescribed for fibromyalgia and MPS are tricyclics, selective serotonin reuptake inhibitors (SSRIs) and serotonin norepinephrine reuptake inhibitors (SNRIs). All of these types of antidepressants have the benefit of being well-studied and so are generally considered safe to use.

The most commonly used tricyclic antidepressant to be used in the treatment of these conditions is amitriptyline, which is usually sold under the brand name of Endep. Other tricyclic antidepressants include desipramine, doxepin, imipramine, amoxapine and nortriptyline which come under a range of different brand names. As the dosages prescribed are usually smaller, the side effects experienced are normally fairly low-level, but can include drowsiness, dizziness, blurred vision, dry mouth, difficulty in urinating, weight gain and sexual dysfunction. Not all patients respond to tricyclics, however, and even in cases where they do, these drugs can lose their effectiveness over time, and sometimes within as little as a month.

Selective serotonin reuptake inhibitors (SSRIs) such as Prozac®, Zoloft®, Paxil® and Luvox® have been shown to improve the chronic fatigue and sleep problems which many fibromyalgia and MPS sufferers experience, as well as promoting a greater sense of general well-being. While some patients claim that they also contribute to the alleviation of pain symptoms, this effect does not seem to apply across the board. The most common side effects of SSRIs are nausea, agitation and sexual dysfunction, including decreased libido and delay in or loss of orgasm. As mentioned previously, SSRIs should not be taken alongside certain painkillers such as tramadol.

SNRIs, or serotonin norepinephrine reuptake inhibitors which are produced under the names of Cymbalta, Effexor and Ixel, act on two chemical messengers in the brain, norepinephrine and serotonin, and in many cases show more consistent benefits than is the case with SSRIs. Cymbalta, an approved drug for the treatment of fibromyalgia, has been shown in certain studies to reduce the pain of the condition by more than 30%, although it can cause side effects such as nausea, dry mouth, decrease in appetite, constipation, sleepiness, increased sweating and agitation. Care should be taken by those patients who are also using non-steroidal anti-inflammatory drugs, aspirin or blood thinners as there could be an increased risk of haemorrhage.

Effexor, which contains venlafaxine, meanwhile, is known to impair sexual function, and there have also been reported cases where patients have experienced changes in blood pressure and where the electrical system of the heart has been affected. These side effects can, of course, be very serious, particularly in the case of elderly patients, although trials have shown that the drug is both safe and effective for the majority of sufferers. On discontinuation of the drug, some people have been known to experience withdrawal symptoms which include nausea and dizziness.

Ixel is another SNRI which many fibromyalgia sufferers report as being highly effective in terms of improving pain symptoms, fatigue and problems with sleep. Many reports from those who have tried the drug suggest that, unlike Cymbalta and Effexor, the side effects in relation to weight gain and sexual issues are much less pronounced or not evident at all. In addition, many claim that Ixel is particularly fast-acting.

Muscle Relaxants

Like antidepressants, muscle relaxants are another group of drugs which have undergone extensive testing and have been found by many sufferers of fibromyalgia and MPS to help alleviate pain symptoms and, in some cases, muscle spasms in particular, although quality of sleep can often improve with the use of these medications too.

Although there are numerous types of muscle relaxant available, the main ones to be used for fibromyalgia and MPS are cyclobenzaprine, orphenadrine citrate, tizanidine and carisoprodol. The different types either work by blocking the transmission of nervous signals to the muscles, so stopping involuntary muscle movement, or by blocking the sensation of pain to the muscles. The taking of muscle relaxants must, however, be carefully overseen, as they can become habit-forming.

Cyclobenzaprine, which is usually sold under the brand name of Flexeril, is one of the varieties of muscle relaxant which blocks the nerve impulses sent from the muscles to the brain, which has the effect of stopping the sensation of pain or stiffness in the muscles. In one study, patients who took the drug also reported a reduction in the number of tender points around the body. Although it has proved to be effective in a good number of cases, however, physicians generally recommend that it only be taken for relatively short periods of time, as longer use can lead to addiction. Being related to the family of tricyclic antidepressants, it also has similar side effects, such as drowsiness, dizziness and dry mouth.

Orphenadrine citrate, meanwhile, also acts on the brain to block muscle pain, but is commonly used alongside physical therapy and rest to achieve maximum effectiveness. As it can be taken for longer periods of time than cyclobenzaprine, it is generally considered to be more effective, with some patients reporting a reduction in pain symptoms of more than 30% after one year of treatment. It can, however, produce some quite disturbing side effects such as tremors and confusion, and so it is important that prolonged use is carefully monitored by a physician. Orphenadrine citrate is marketed under the name of Norflex.

Tizanidine is a particularly useful drug for individuals who suffer not only from pain symptoms, but also from muscle spasms. Working again to block the nerve impulses which are carried to the brain, it is, in fact, one of the most effective medications for muscle spasms and also carries the benefit of improving muscle tone and reducing weakness. Marketed under the trade name of Zanaflex, tizanidine is not suitable for patients who either suffer from liver or kidney disease or are taking oral contraceptives. Constipation, dizziness, drowsiness, flushing and dry mouth are some of the most common side effects of this drug.

The drug known as carisoprodol, which is sold under the brand name of Soma, although less well-studied than the other types of muscle relaxant, has also shown excellent results in terms of reducing muscle spasms, as well as muscle pain and stiffness. Its most common side effects are dizziness, drowsiness and headaches.

Benzodiazepines

The prescription of benzodiazepines such as Diazepam, Temazepam, Clonazepam and Triazolam is frequently avoided by many doctors, or at least if they are prescribed it is generally only for short periods of time, as dependency can become a real issue. Benzodiazepines, which have a hypnotic and sedative effect can, however, be beneficial in terms of relaxing tense, painful muscles and dealing with insomnia, and have also been found to be effective where restless leg syndrome is one of the related medical problems experienced. The side effect of these psychotropic drugs may include depression, memory impairment, blurred vision, confusion, impaired co-ordination, trembling, change in heart rate, weakness and an increase in the number of dreams or nightmares.

Sleep Medications

Although insomnia and disturbed sleep patterns can affect sufferers of both fibromyalgia and MPS, it is generally those with fibromyalgia who experience greater problems and who suffer from the chronic fatigue which impacts so considerably on their daily lives. While the use of some pain relievers, anti-convulsants, antidepressants and muscle relaxants can bring about better quality of sleep, sometimes it is necessary for doctors to prescribe medications which are specifically designed to bring about more restful sleep.

Benzodiazepines such as those noted previously are sometimes prescribed for their sedative qualities, although as mentioned, longer term use does not come without the risk of addiction. While imidazopyridines, such as zolpidem, zopiclone and zalepon, act on the same receptors in the brain as benzodiazepines, they are, however, less likely to cause addiction, but should still only be taken on a short-term basis. The side effects associated with this group of drugs commonly include nausea, dizziness, vertigo, nightmares and skin rashes.

Barbiturates work by suppressing the activity in the central nervous system, so aiding more restful sleep. They also, however, help to inhibit nerve and muscle activity, which not only limits pain, but also contributes to the quality of sleep by reducing muscle twitches and spasms. Phenobarbital is probably one of the most well-known barbiturates, although there are numerous others available on the market too. As with benzodiazepines, many doctors will avoid prescribing barbiturates because of the potential for addiction. In addition, one of the side effects of these drugs is that they can cause muscle and joint pain, as well as fever, sore throats, wheezing, chest pain, swollen eyelids and face and skin problems.

Most commonly used to relieve allergy and cold symptoms, antihistamines can also be taken as a sleeping aid because they induce drowsiness. As they can cause side effects such as dizziness, blurred vision, dry mouth and confusion, however, anyone buying these medications over the counter should be aware that they should only be used on a short-term basis.

24

Pain Reduction Methods

As well as the wide range of medications which are aimed at alleviating the symptoms of fibromyalgia and MPS, there are also a variety of traditional and alternative therapies which some sufferers have found to be effective, specifically in terms of relieving their pain. In this chapter, we will be looking at some of these options, which could prove to be beneficial either as an alternative to traditional medication or which might be used as a complement to it. It is important to remember, however, that finding an experienced medical professional to carry out these treatments is vital if significant relief is to be achieved and further problems avoided.

Massage Therapy

Massage therapy has been around for centuries and has been used throughout the ages to help with a whole range of physical and psychological ailments. When carried out by a trained practitioner who not only understands the technique itself, but is also knowledgeable about the conditions that he or she is treating, it can be considered as a safe and effective method of pain relief.

There are various types of massage therapy which can help to relieve the pain experienced by sufferers of fibromyalgia and MPS, but what they all have in common is the fact that they 'attack' the pain in more than one way. First of all, they work directly on the muscles to release the tension within them and alleviate the feeling of stiffness; but in addition, of course, massage is an excellent way to promote relaxation and drive away the stress which can very easily contribute to troublesome symptoms. The incidence and the levels of anxiety and depression in those who regularly receive massage therapy have also been found to be lower than in those who do not, and sleep problems have additionally been shown to improve as a result. In fact, for many fibromyalgia and MPS patients, massage therapy is considered to be one of the most beneficial treatments.

Most types of massage therapy involve the manipulation of the muscles and soft tissues of the body using the hands. In some cases, a kneading action might be used, whilst in others it might be stroking or palpation. In others still, massage might also be combined with hot and cold therapies to help increase the blood flow to the muscles or to relax them.

Two of the most commonly used massage therapies which have proved to be beneficial for fibromyalgia sufferers are Swedish massage and deep tissue massage, while many MPS patients have experienced great success with trigger point therapy. Myofascial release techniques, meanwhile, have been found by many to provide relief for both conditions.

Swedish Massage

The first of these, Swedish massage, is a gentle form of massage which is nevertheless deep enough to be effective in reducing pain levels. The technique is aimed at increasing the amount of oxygen to the muscles and not only helps to improve their flexibility, but also their general health and ability to repair themselves. Swedish massage mainly involves using the thumbs, fingertips and palms of the hands to stroke the body in long, gliding movements, although tapping and kneading may also form part of the therapy, which also involves vibration techniques.

Deep Tissue Massage

Deep tissue massage, on the other hand, is a more vigorous form of therapy which involves making slow, deep and pressurised strokes either along or across the muscles. Although ultimately more effective at loosening areas of hard or inflexible muscle and tissue and relieving chronic pain, patients do sometimes experience some discomfort for a day or so immediately following the treatment.

Trigger Point Therapy

Another form of treatment for pain which is similar to massage therapy is trigger point therapy. Although designed to alleviate the pain emanating from the trigger points of MPS sufferers, and despite the slightly confusing terminology (remember that trigger points refer pain to other sites in the body and are not the same as the tender points associated with fibromyalgia), trigger point therapy can be highly effective for sufferers of both fibromyalgia and MPS, as well as for those with other chronic pain disorders. In the case of MPS it is the trigger points which are worked on and, in the case of fibromyalgia, the tender points.

The aim of trigger point therapy is to work directly on the tender and hyperirritable spots in the body which cause localised or referred pain, by eliminating tender points or deactivating trigger points. It involves locating the relevant points on the body (which can be as small as a pinhead and are only rarely the size of a thumb knuckle) and applying continual pressure to them for around 10 seconds using the fingers, knuckles or elbows, releasing and then following up with a further 30 seconds or so of pressure in a pumping action. Because the tender or trigger points are painful in themselves, manipulating them in this way is bound to cause some degree of pain or discomfort, although most people describe the pain as being 'pleasant' and not at a level which causes the body to tense up.

Trigger point therapy is not an instant cure and, particularly in cases where trigger points have been active for some years, it can take a few months to deactivate them. In addition, it is important to find an expert in this technique because if the pressure is applied for too short a time, deactivation of the trigger point will not occur and, if applied too hard or for too long, it can irritate the point even further or cause painful bruising which can last for up to three days afterwards.

Myofascial Release Techniques

Myofascial release techniques are designed to work on the muscle fascia, the thin layer of tissue which covers all the muscles and organs of the body. The aim of the treatment is to stretch the fascia which, in both fibromyalgia and MPS sufferers may have become short and tense, so that relief from stiffness and pain is experienced.

To do this, the therapist will use a variety of stretching and skin rolling techniques. After having located the areas where the body feels tight and stiff, he or she will gradually stretch the area, hold the stretch and then allow the muscle fascia to relax, repeating the process until full muscle relaxation is achieved.

Myofascial release is quite commonly used in cases where the patient has suffered a whiplash injury prior to the onset of fibromyalgia or MPS, and is often used in conjunction with trigger point therapy to focus on the area of trigger or tender points.

Craniosacral Therapy

Craniosacral therapy is considered by some to be a form of myofascial release technique, but instead of working directly on the fascia of the muscles throughout the body, it concentrates on the skull and the spine. By tuning in to the natural rhythms of the body and working with the tiny movements of the bones in the head, it is believed that the therapy can affect the whole of the central nervous system by removing restrictions in the nerve passages and promoting the body's ability to heal itself. The therapy uses an extremely light touch and is so gentle and relaxing that it can be used on patients of any age, including very young babies.

Physical Therapy

Although massage therapy in itself is a form of physical therapy, there are also other types of physical therapy which can help fibromyalgia and MPS sufferers to gain some relief from their pain, as well as to increase their strength and mobility. Physical therapists work with their patients to teach them ways in which they can help themselves, such as by showing them how to do stretching and other types of exercise which will help to alleviate their symptoms and prevent painful flare-ups from occurring. In addition, trained therapists who have studied in the areas of anatomy and kinesiology (the study of movement) will also ensure that your posture and movement are correct, so that your muscles can function effectively and further problems are not allowed to develop. The programmes that they design are tailor-made to suit the individual needs of each and every patient.

Hydrotherapy

Hydrotherapy is another ancient therapy, but this time it involves the use of water, either internally or externally, to treat illness or injury or to maintain sound health. Since ancient Roman times, people have visited spas to help relieve them of their aches and pains, and even today water therapy is still very popular.

Hydrotherapy might involve being totally immersed in water and carrying out gentle aerobic exercises. Being in a gravity-free environment, patients are often able to perform exercises which, on dry land, might otherwise be extremely difficult or painful for them to manage. In other cases, however, hydrotherapy might use moist heat or cold packs applied to the surface of the body to achieve pain relief. Warm, moist compresses which are placed on painful areas of the body, for example, help to dilate the blood vessels so that the flow of blood, oxygen and other nutrients is increased, and can be a very effective way of reducing and managing pain.

Waon therapy, which might be considered to be a form of hydro-therapy, has been shown to provide significant pain relief for some fibromyalgia patients. This involves sitting first of all in a dry sauna and then being wrapped in blankets and being placed in a warm room.

Trigger Point Injections

Like trigger point therapy, trigger point injections were designed to deal mainly with the painful symptoms experienced by sufferers of MPS. In some cases, however, they have also proved to be equally effective for releasing the tight muscle knots which those with fibro-myalgia will be very familiar with. Generally, trigger point injections will only be used on particularly painful tender points and, although there may be some pain and bruising for a day or two after the treat-ment, sustained relief lasting for two to three months can often be achieved after only a brief course of injections.

The procedure for administering trigger point injections involves the physician inserting a needle into and around the affected trigger or tender points in the body. In some cases, the injection may contain nothing more than saline solution, whilst in others the doctor may use a very small amount of a local anaesthetic such as lidocaine or procaine to numb the area, and sometimes a corticosteroid may also be used to help relieve pain. Once the liquid has been injected, the trigger or tender point will then be massaged for several minutes.

In some cases, patients who undergo trigger point injections experience soreness or bruising for several days afterwards, and even increased levels of pain, but this is then typically followed by a significant reduction in symptoms. In other cases, sufferers experience almost immediate relief. The application of heat or cold and carrying out stretching exercises can help considerably in the meantime with any post-injection pain or discomfort.

Botox

Although botox is most commonly thought of in relation to cosmetic procedures designed to reduce the effects of wrinkling, it is also used to help with the symptoms of a number of illnesses such as multiple sclerosis and cerebral palsy, and has also been found to be useful for stroke victims. In relation to easing the pain and spasms associated with fibromyalgia and MPS, it is fast becoming thought of as a 'miracle cure' however.

Botox is basically a drug made from a toxin produced by the bacterium Clostridium botulinum, which is purified before being used for cosmetic or medical purposes. When administered in small doses, it has the effect of blocking neuromuscular transmission and causing selective weakening and paralysis of muscles, thereby alleviating pain and spasms. Used firstly and with great effect on patients suffering from MPS to target the trigger points in the affected muscles, botox is now being used to help fibromyalgia sufferers too.

In one study which was carried out by the Pain Evaluation and Treatment Center in Tulsa, USA, 70% of MPS sufferers who experienced pain in the back and extremities reported a very significant reduction in symptoms for between two and four months are receiving botox injections over a two-year period. Reports in relation to its use with fibromyalgia sufferers are showing equally favourable results.

The procedure for administering botox is perfectly safe, since only small amounts of the drug are used, but it does need to be administered by a trained specialist. Rarely are there any after-effects and even then these are only comparable to flu-like symptoms. It should also be noted that frequent injections can lead to an immunity to the drug. Where there is an underlying medical condition other than fibromyalgia or MPS, it may not be possible for patients to receive botox injections, but this is something which your pain consultant should be able to advise you on.

The effects of botox injections typically take between one and three weeks to become evident, but may then last for up to four months.

Acupuncture

Acupuncture is a procedure in which fine needles are inserted into the skin at specific points to relieve pain or for other therapeutic purposes. It has been used for centuries, although how it first came to be used and how its benefits were first discovered are uncertain. As the theory on how it works is concerned with adjusting the life energy which is believed to flow through us all and is not grounded in any scientific principle, some scientists and physicians are sceptical about its use. Despite this, however, patients suffering from a whole range of painful illnesses and injuries have found that it has helped them to achieve at least an element of relief.

Both traditional Chinese acupuncture and electroacupuncture, the latter of which involves the doctor or therapist attaching clips to the needles so that a continuous electrical impulse stimulates the acupuncture point, are very popular with fibromyalgia and MPS patients. Although wider studies into the effectiveness of these techniques in sufferers of these conditions are somewhat limited, many individuals find that they experience temporary relief from pain symptoms, although problems with chronic fatigue, sleep problems and physical function are not normally improved. Where patients suffer from adverse reactions to traditional forms of medication, acupuncture may offer at least some relief from pain.

While most acupuncture therapists are believed to produce good results in terms of treatment, of course great care needs to be taken in choosing a reputable acupuncturist who uses sterile needles in order to protect your own personal safety. It should also be noted that patients who use medications which are intended to thin the blood, or who have any type of bleeding disorders, may not be suitable for acupuncture therapy.

Intramuscular Stimulation

Intramuscular stimulation (IMS) is a dry needling method of treatment which is similar to acupuncture but is based more around scientific principles. In this case, when a tiny needle is inserted into the skin, the tight, contracted muscle grabs hold of it and then, after a while, relaxes. Rather than contracting again immediately after the needle is withdrawn, the muscle stays relaxed long afterwards, thus providing considerable relief from pain for many of those with fibromyalgia and MPS. In some cases the needle may be manipulated whilst it is still sticking into the skin, while in others a small amount of vibration might be introduced or a mild electrical current applied to achieve an even greater effect.

Chiropractic/Osteopathic Manipulation

Although some patients have reported decreased pain levels and improved sleep as a result of chiropractic or osteopathic manipulation, great care needs to be taken with either of these techniques. Where the spine or the neck in particular is being manipulated, damage to the body can be inflicted, and in rare cases patients have even suffered a stroke as a result.

Case Study 1

Tender point (trigger point) in the thigh successfully treated with local injection of cortisone and pulsed radiofrequency

A 42-year-old gentleman was found to have a specific tender point on the right medial part of the thigh at the top, which was believed to be a localised area of inflammation of tendon or local inflamed muscle. He had had some benefit from non-steroidal anti-inflammatories but, unfortunately, this was only short-lived.

The gentleman was brought into the clinic and the area was injected with 1 ml of 0.5% Bupivacaine and 80 mg of Depo-Medrone steroid. This gave him good relief for around three months, at which time the procedure was repeated, which again provided good relief for a further three months.

As the patient was very keen not to take any further medication, but preferred to find a more long-term solution, pulsed radiofrequency was applied locally to the area with 80 mg Depo-Medrone steroid. He was seen four months later in the Pain Clinic and was still found to be experiencing a good degree of pain relief and so was discharged.

Case Study 2

Myofascial pain syndrome treated with local anaesthetic and anti-inflammatory medication

A 77-year-old man who was seen in the Pain Clinic was experiencing pain in his neck and lower back (L3/L4 region), as well as in areas over the trapezius muscles of the shoulders. He also had some difficulty in swallowing and was taking only small quantities of food. The pain was described as a dull ache with an average score of 5/10. The pain, which came and went, was very localised with no radiations and no pins and needles. It was aggravated by eating and the movement of his arm, and relieved by lying flat. What was particularly notable was the fact that since 1985 he had suffered from spondylosis (narrowing) of the cervical spine.

Drug history: Paracetamol or paracetamol and codeine combinations

Past medical history:

- Temporal arthritis
- Cervical spondylosis
- Insulin-dependent diabetes
- Angina
- Intermittent shortness of breath

On examination, the gentleman's head was held in an extremely flexed position with a fixed cervical flexion deformity noted at the C7/T1 level. On palpation, there were multiple trigger points in the neck, in the trapezius muscles, the rhomboid muscles and over the shoulders and back area. These trigger points gave pain on deep palpation. The impression was of MPS, secondary to chronic cervical spondylolysthesis.

Management plan: The initial plan for the gentleman was to start with a conservative management which included deep tissue massage and a course of 6–10 acupuncture sessions.

Medication: Amitriptyline or Gabapentin in small doses.

More invasive treatments: Local anaesthetic and steroid injections or Botulinum Toxin (botox) injections to local trigger points.

Rehabilitation: Physiotherapy in order to change his posture and training regarding posture.

As the gentleman was not keen on medication, over the course of two weeks he received daily acupuncture for 10 days and local injections (wet needling) to trigger points with local anaesthesia and steroid. His symptoms subsided during the course of treatment, after which time he returned to his home abroad.

Case Study 3

Fibromyalgia treated with acupuncture and injection of local anaesthetic and anti-inflammatory

I saw a 60-year-old lady in the Pain Clinic with all over body pain, including pain in the neck, hip, leg, shoulders and lower back. On examination, she had a number of trigger points on her back and there was also a reduction on internal and external rotation and flexion and extension of her hip joints. Both hip joints were painful on palpation.

In the first instance, the lady was not keen on taking medication and instead opted for a course of six acupuncture treatments which she had at 1–2 weekly intervals. At the end of this course of treatment, she found that both her sleep and her pain had improved.

Although she had previously been taking amitriptyline 25 mg at night, she decided to stop this. After approximately one month, however, she found that the pain was beginning to return and so decided to opt for medication once again. She was started on Gabapentin 300 mg three times daily, which was increased to 500 mg three times a day. At this higher dose though, she began to experience a number of adverse effects, including tiredness, dizziness and a lack of energy. The dose was therefore reduced back down to 400 mg three times a day.

Two months later, the lady found that her pain was worsening again but she was not keen to increase the dosage of medication. The next step, therefore, was to perform injections of local anaesthetic and steroid into the trigger points. This was done on an outpatient basis using aseptic technique with gloves, gown and chlorhexidine. A total of 20 trigger points in the back, neck and shoulders were injected with approximately 1 ml of solution to a total of 20 mls of 0.5% Bupivacaine, local anaesthetic and 80 mg of Depo-Medrone steroid.

When the lady's condition was reviewed two months later, she reported great benefit from the wet needling and a dramatic reduction in her pain scores. She was now only taking Gabepentin 300 mg at night, which she had arranged for herself. We agreed to discharge her from the clinic and see her again should her symptoms return.

25

Alternative Remedies and Treatments

Although there are those physicians who still prefer to stick rigidly with more traditional treatments, not just for fibromyalgia and MPS, but also for many other illnesses and injuries, more and more are accepting of alternative and complementary treatments too. Quite commonly, it is because the effectiveness of alternative treatments is not supported by scientific studies or evidence which turns those in the medical professions off them, but as so many people seem to gain such benefit from them, increasing numbers of doctors are quite happy to recommend their use as part of a holistic treatment programme.

Ideally, you should work with a practitioner who uses both traditional and alternative and complementary techniques, so that he or she can monitor the impact of one type of treatment or therapy against any others which are being used. Certain herbal supplements, for example, although widely available and purporting to be effective for fibromyalgia and MPS symptoms, might interfere with the effectiveness of more traditional medications, so it is important that your doctor has a full overview of the treatments being used and/or prescribed.

Some of the most popular alternative and complementary treatments used by fibromyalgia and MPS sufferers are herbal remedies, supplements and natural remedies, and here we are going to take a quick look at each.

Herbal and Other Natural Remedies

Herbal and other natural remedies have been used by our ancestors since time immemorial and are still very popular with many people today. Although, just like traditional medications, they cannot cure fibromyalgia or MPS, some patients do find that they provide relief from certain of their symptoms. Here are some of the main ones to consider:

- **Ginger** – Whether you use ginger in its natural form, take it in the form of ginger tea or swallow ginger capsules, this root offers a range of therapeutic benefits including relief from muscle aches and pains, as well as from the nausea and headaches which sufferers sometimes experience.
- **Turmeric** – Turmeric contains a powerful anti-inflammatory ingredient which is excellent for treating muscle pain and, in addition, it helps to rid the body of dangerous toxins.
- **Gotu kola** – Used in India for its medicinal properties for thousands of years, this plant helps to strengthen tissues and blood vessels, as well as having rejuvenating and anti-inflammatory properties.
- **Cayenne** – Many herbalists consider cayenne to be the most valuable herb of all. Rich in vitamins A, B and C, it is also high in organic calcium and potassium, making it extremely good for the heart and the digestive and circulatory systems. In terms of fibromyalgia and MPS, it can be very effective at reducing pain.
- **Chaparral** – This scrubland plant is known as an anti-inflammatory of the intestinal tissue which also helps to calm nerve endings.
- **Horsetail** – This relative of the fern not only helps to strengthen the nails, hair and bones, but also the connective tissues of the body.
- **Nettle** – The nettle is excellent for helping you to build up energy and for stimulating the metabolism.
- **Willow** – White willow bark in particular has been found by many to be especially effective in dealing with muscle pain and fever. In fact, it has been shown to be every bit as effective as aspirin, but rarely has any side effects.
- **Ginseng** – Like nettle, ginseng is also great for building up energy levels and stimulating the metabolism.
- **Valerian** – Valerian root is a natural relaxant and helps greatly in achieving more restful and restorative sleep. In addition, it can help those who are anxious or tense to relax more during the course of the day.

With any herbal or natural remedy, it is important to remember that you may still suffer side effects in just the same way as you might if you were taking more traditional forms of medication. In addition, some may be harmful to people with other conditions or to women who are pregnant or breastfeeding.

Supplements

Poor diets and illness in particular can leave our bodies deficient in essential vitamins and minerals, and these deficiencies in turn can cause additional problems. In most people's lives there are times when they need a top-up of one kind or another and, in the case of fibromyalgia and MPS patients, certain types of supplements have proved to be beneficial.

Magnesium

Of all the deficiencies to have been detected in fibromyalgia and MPS sufferers, as well as in patients suffering from chronic fatigue syndrome, magnesium is one of the most common. Responsible for supporting a healthy immune system, regulating the heartbeat, keeping bones healthy and strong, helping to regulate blood sugar levels and keep blood pressure at a normal level, magnesium is required for more than 300 biochemical reactions to take place in the body. When we are in pain or are suffering from stress, however, essential magnesium is lost from the kidneys through the urine, which almost certainly accounts for why so many sufferers of chronic pain are found to be deficient.

The symptoms of magnesium deficiency are many, but interestingly, a good few of them are shared with those of fibromyalgia and MPS. Muscle spasms, cramps and weakness, insomnia and fatigue, confusion, nausea, anxiety and irritability, diarrhoea and other symptoms of irritable bowel syndrome can all show up in people with magnesium deficiency, but are also very common symptoms of fibromyalgia and MPS. In addition, those with insufficient levels of magnesium have also been found to be more vulnerable to stressful stimuli such as loud noise and chemical smells, which of course is something else which is commonly found in fibromyalgia sufferers in particular.

Those diagnosed with fibromyalgia and MPS are well-advised, therefore, to have their magnesium levels checked by their physicians and to take supplements if appropriate.

Vitamins

Although some studies have shown sufferers of fibromyalgia and MPS to be deficient in vitamins B1 and E, it is low levels of vitamin D which have caused most excitement amongst scientists in relation to these two conditions. Although it seems highly unlikely that vitamin D deficiency is the sole cause of the illnesses, some research appears to indicate that it could be a factor in the development or the aggravation of the conditions, and in particular the muscular pain and weakness which is associated with them.

The way in which vitamin D is believed to be relevant to the onset or progression of fibromyalgia is this. The body contains a hormone known as parathyroid hormone, which is responsible for extracting phosphates, and especially calcium phosphate, from the bones. Vitamin D deficiency essentially depletes the body of parathyroid hormone, so that there are abnormally high levels of phosphate retained in the bones, and it is this which might account for the as yet unexplained bone and muscle pain which fibromyalgia patients experience.

Although vitamin D is contained in a small number of foods such as oily fish, eggs, margarine, breakfast cereals and powdered milk, most of our exposure to it comes from sunlight. Whilst there are, of course, other dangers associated with prolonged exposure to sunlight, our bodies do need some exposure in order to remain healthy and to keep our levels of vitamin D topped up.

Omega-3

The human body requires two main types of essential fatty acids, known as omega-6 and omega-3, in order to remain healthy. Omega-6 comes from corn, sunflower, soy and other types of oil, whilst omega-3 is found in fish oil, but in relatively few other food-stuffs. Our bodies cannot make either of these fatty acids, so the only way that we can maintain sufficient levels is through our diet or by taking supplements. Years ago, the balance of omega-6 to omega-3 was thought to be at a ratio of 1:1, but the changes in our diet now mean that in some cases it can be more like 20:1 or even 50:1 and consequently a huge proportion of the population is believed to be highly deficient in omega-3.

Omega-3 plays a number of very important roles in the body, not least in protecting us from the risk of heart disease, arthritis, depression and certain types of cancer to name but a few. A deficiency, however, has been associated with a number of illnesses and disorders, of which fibromyalgia is just one.

Acetyl-L-Carnitine

Acetyl-L-carnitine occurs naturally in plants and animals and can be taken as a dietary supplement. It is typically recommended to improve the memory of those who suffer from Alzheimer's disease, to help with depression, for those diagnosed with Parkinson's disease and for those who have suffered a stroke. In one study, however, supplementation of acetyl-L-carnitine for a period of ten weeks was shown to significantly improve the musculoskeletal pain, depression and general health of fibromyalgia patients.

Serotonin

The hormone serotonin, which acts as a chemical messenger to transmit nerve signals, is essential for normal nerve and brain function but has often been found to exist in only low levels in sufferers of fibromyalgia. The substance known as 5-Hydroxytryptophan or 5-HTP is used by the body to make serotonin but is not present in significant amounts in the normal diet. In the case of fibromyalgia sufferers with low serotonin levels, supplementation with 5-HTP has been found through a number of trials to relieve some of the symptoms of the condition.

Melatonin

Melatonin, which is another natural hormone, is associated with the sleep–wake cycle, which of course is often very much disturbed in patients suffering from fibromyalgia and MPS. A preliminary trial which was conducted on fibromyalgia patients showed that melatonin supplementation given at bedtime reduced tender points and improved sleep, although improvements in terms of pain and fatigue were only slight.

S-adenosylmethionine

S-adenosylmethionine (SAMe) is a compound which occurs naturally in almost every tissue and fluid in the human body and is associated with many important processes. Not only does it play a role in the effective functioning of the immune system, but it also maintains cell membranes and helps to produce and break down brain chemicals such as serotonin, melatonin and dopamine. Because it works with vitamins B12 and B6, low levels of these vitamins can also reduce the levels of SAMe.

Numerous scientific studies have been carried out in relation to SAMe, particularly with regard to osteoarthritis and depression, and have shown that supplementation can have quite considerable effects. Given orally over a period of six weeks, several trials with fibromyalgia sufferers saw significant reductions in levels of pain, fatigue and stiffness, as well as improving the overall mood of the sufferers.

As is the case with herbal remedies, natural supplements can have negative side effects as well as positive effects, and so it is extremely important that you consult with a doctor before using any of these.

26

Cognitive Behavioural Therapy

The methods for managing and controlling the symptoms of fibromyalgia and MPS that we have looked at in the previous three chapters have, of course, all revolved around taking different types of medications or supplements, or taking part in different types of physical therapies. Cognitive behavioural therapy (CBT), however, represents a completely different approach to the conditions, but has still been shown to reduce the severity of symptoms while at the same time improving patients' quality of life.

As was described earlier in this book, dealing effectively with chronic conditions such as fibromyalgia and MPS requires a multi-pronged approach. While the prescription of traditional forms of medication, the use of supplements or taking part in physical therapy might each in themselves have some impact on the severity of the conditions, it is generally when a combination of different treatments is applied that the sufferer experiences greatest relief.

One of the biggest problems with any kind of chronic illness, however, is that it not only affects the body, but also the mind, often leading sufferers to develop a strong sense of negativity and a range of self-defeating behaviours. What CBT does is to help patients to replace these unhelpful thoughts, feelings and behaviours with ones which are much more constructive and positive. The consequent increase in the sense of control over their lives that they feel, and the reduction in their levels of stress can, in turn, have positive benefits in relation to their physical symptoms.

Cognitive behavioural therapy is a 'talk' treatment, but unlike many other types of talk therapy which delve way back into patients' pasts, it concentrates on the problems that they are experiencing in the here and now and seeks to address them. Essentially, it helps to change how the patient thinks (cognitive) and how they act (behaviour) so that they can cope better. It is a therapy which is used to help patients who are suffering from a whole range of chronic illnesses, including rheumatoid arthritis and cancer, and has been shown to be very effective in cases involving fibromyalgia and MPS.

Although it may not feel this way a lot of the time, our emotions are something over which we have control, in just the same way as our behaviour. When we become more aware of thoughts and feelings which are ultimately self-defeating, then we can make a conscious decision to change them, and this is what CBT sets out to achieve. To give just one example of how this might apply, think of all the times when you, the sufferer, have felt angry and frustrated by the limitations of your illness, so angry and frustrated in fact that you then went on to push yourself to your limits. The result, I would be prepared to bet, was that not only did your physical symptoms flare up, but you felt on the point of mental breakdown too. Being then unable to cope with even the simplest of tasks, you probably felt even more demoralised and unworthy and just felt like giving up – and my bet is that this has happened not dozens of times, but hundreds. By helping you to define and set realistic limits and teaching you how to say 'No' and be comfortable with that, CBT can mean avoiding this vicious circle and so can ultimately make your life more manageable.

The stress and anxiety that we experience as a result of feelings of helplessness, hopelessness, self-loathing and so on are immensely damaging to us in both a psychological and physical sense, and unless sufferers of fibromyalgia and MPS learn how to reverse these negative trends it is all too easy to spiral down into depression and to cause physical symptoms to worsen. By taking conscious control of managing their pain, learning to cope with their changed lives and with stressful situations, as well as learning how to relax, however, the destructive forces can be reversed.

27

Lifestyle Changes

Discovering that you have a chronic condition for which there is no known cause or cure and accepting it are, of course, two completely different things. Without acceptance, however, there is no possibility of incorporating change into your life, and chronic illnesses, almost without exception, require that change be made.

I am quite sure that for many of those who are reading this, the very prospect of changing your lifestyle is a terrifying one. In fact, for the vast, vast majority of people, change of any kind and in any area of their lives fills them with dread, and yet in reality we humans are incredibly adaptable and resourceful. We marry, we have children, we move house and change cars and jobs, sometimes we divorce and remarry, our children leave home and we learn to cope when we lose those who are close to us.

Even in our daily lives we face endless changes. We might replace an old tool or piece of kitchen equipment with a new model, but we learn how to operate it and, within no time at all, it feels like an old friend. Our offices undergo reorganisations and we have to change position and sit beside a complete stranger, and not only do we cope, but very soon we cannot even remember what things were like before. Our local supermarket changes hands and the first time we visit we might become frustrated because we can't find anything, but by the third or fourth trip, we know that the shampoos are in aisle four and frozen chickens in aisle ten.

No matter whether the changes that you have faced in your life have been as a matter of your own choice or whether they have been imposed on you, and no matter how much you tell yourself that you hate change, I guarantee that you are an expert in dealing with it. Granted, some of you will have dealt with it more easily than others, but the ease with which you handled it will almost certainly be in direct proportion to your acceptance that it either needed to happen or was inevitable.

If you have already been diagnosed with fibromyalgia or MPS, the chances are that your lifestyle has already changed in the time that it has taken to diagnose your condition. In your struggle to cope with the agonising pain, the chronic fatigue and sleepless nights, as well as a whole range of other debilitating and sometimes frightening symptoms, you will at the very least have cried off a few engagements or taken a lie down when you might otherwise have been doing something fun or constructive. In all likelihood though, you did those things with feelings of anger, bitterness, regret or guilt, and you are probably still beating yourself up for them now.

When we make changes consciously in our lives, they are much, much easier to accept than otherwise. In the case of chronic illnesses, when we accept that change is necessary and inevitable, we are left feeling that we are the ones who are in control, not the condition, and so living with it becomes very much easier. It is not a case of giving in to the illness or of giving up, but of taking back the control of our own lives, and in many cases all it takes is to establish some new routines, something which the hard-wiring of our brains makes not only entirely possible, but also relatively easy.

In the course of the next few chapters, we are going to look at some of the more major adaptations that sufferers of fibromyalgia and MPS can make to ensure a more comfortable and better quality life. These include topics such as diet, exercise, posture, sleep and dealing with stress. For the remainder of this chapter, however, I want to indicate a few more general things that you can do to improve your day-to-day situation.

Time yourself

Because fibromyalgia and MPS can often be triggered by repetitive motions or the prolonged tensing of muscles, it is important not to keep going at one single activity for too long. Try setting a stop watch or alarm to go off every 20 minutes, and then when it does, stop what you are doing and do something else for a few minutes. For example, if you were sitting at the computer, get up and take a short walk.

Pace yourself

Typically, those who suffer from fibromyalgia or MPS have good days and bad days. Because the bad days can sometimes leave them unable to do very much at all, they try to cram as much as possible into the good days in order to catch up or get ahead. Actually though, this works against you, because the good days are then quite likely to be followed by several days in which your condition feels even worse. Try, therefore, to pace yourself and keep your activity level the same each day.

Rest

Remember to take regular rest breaks. You may not have needed to do so in the past, but avoiding it now is only likely to lead to an increase in flare-ups and bad days.

Write things down

The confusion and mental fog which is commonly experienced by sufferers of fibromyalgia can leave them feeling as though they are losing their minds, which of course they are not. Rather than beating yourself up about the fact that you cannot remember things as well as you used to, give yourself a break and write them down.

A place for everything

For the same reasons as above, find a place for everything and always return things to their rightful place. In this way, you are less likely to be left scratching your head if you are having a bad day and your memory is failing you.

De-clutter

Trying to get through even simple tasks like housework can feel all the more impossible when you are surrounded by clutter. Without doing it all at once and exhausting yourself, gradually get rid of the clutter so that things are easier to do and easier to find. Even something as simple as clearing away some of the ornaments that you normally keep on show will make dusting quicker and easier.

Reorganise if necessary

Look around your home and see what you can do to rearrange furniture, cupboards and so on to make life easier. If there are things that you use regularly which are currently in high cupboards which you now find difficult to reach, then put them somewhere lower. If your favourite armchair is currently placed beside a draughty window and the draught causes your symptoms to flare up, then move it somewhere warmer.

Prioritise
Again, with both good days and bad days to face, managing your time to fit in everything that you either must do or want to do is vital if frustration, anxiety and depression are to be avoided. Accept that you cannot do everything and then prioritise your tasks, focusing on the doable and not the impossible.

Give yourself enough time
What may have taken you five minutes in the past might, on an average day, now take considerably longer. Factor in extra time so that you do not have to over-exert yourself or rush to get things done.

Avoid your own stressors
Different things cause stress to different people. Work out what stresses you and then avoid these things as much as you possibly can, especially if you are going through a particularly rough spell. Not only will this benefit your mental health, but your physical health too.

28

Diet

While no-one would dispute the fact that eating a healthy diet is crucial for fibromyalgia and MPS sufferers, unfortunately there is no single diet which will bring about improvements to all. Because the conditions can encompass such a huge range of symptoms which are experienced to varying degrees by different individuals, what works for one person may have completely the opposite effect on another. Having said this, however, there are some foodstuffs which are generally considered to be more or less beneficial than others.

Keeping a Food Journal

Before we go on to take a look at specific types of food and drink and the effects that they might have on fibromyalgia and MPS symptoms, I just want to take a moment to mention the benefits of keeping a food diary.

A great many people who suffer from these two conditions find that certain foods make them feel worse, but trying to pinpoint precisely what is causing the problem when your diet might contain any number of different foods and drinks can be tricky. By keeping a diary of what you eat on each day, and also noting any flare-ups in your various symptoms, you can more easily identify which elements of your diet, if any, are contributing to these. Remember though to pay attention to all of your symptoms, such as pain levels, headaches or migraines, constipation and diarrhoea and so on, because even being able to alleviate one of these could improve your quality of life considerably.

It does not matter how you keep your diary – it could be in a notebook or on an Excel spreadsheet or whatever you find most convenient – but what is important is that you keep it up to date. Whether you are eating at home, at a friend's house or in a restaurant, note down everything you eat, every time you eat.

The Elimination Diet

Another way to try and establish whether certain foodstuffs or drinks are contributing to or causing a worsening of your symptoms is to try the elimination diet. Although it might sound fairly drastic, all it involves is cutting out certain elements of your diet and then reintroducing them one at a time to see what effect it has.

To begin with, try eliminating broad categories of foods – you might, for example, start with dairy products – and then one by one, reintroduce milk, butter and so on and see how you feel. If none of the foods in this particular category appear to make any difference, then start again, but eliminate, for example, wheat-based products instead.

Of course, at the same time as carrying out the elimination diet, you will also need to maintain your food diary, otherwise remembering what you have cut out or reintroduced on any one day could become a huge challenge. In addition, try to time your diet so that it does not coincide with periods of high stress, flare-ups or holidays during which you might be eating completely different kinds of food.

Problem Foodstuffs

As we have said, what may be a problem in terms of foodstuffs for you, may have no effect on another sufferer of fibromyalgia or MPS, but there are certain categories of food which, when cut out altogether or cut back on, do seem to have greater effect, not just in terms of improving a whole range of symptoms, but also general levels of health, vitality and weight, and these include:

- Refined sugar
- Red meat
- Polyunsaturated vegetable oils
- Margarine
- Vegetable shortening
- Foods which are high in starch such as bread and potatoes
- Chocolate
- All deep-fried foods

- Any highly processed foods
- Any foods containing monosodium glutamate (MSG) or MSG plus aspartame

In the case of the latter, one albeit very limited study showed that women who eliminated MSG or MSG and aspartame from their diets experienced either a marked improvement in their conditions or their symptoms disappeared altogether. In each case, the symptoms returned every time that MSG was reintroduced into their diet.

As well as these foodstuffs, caffeine, alcohol and fizzy drinks have also proved to cause problems for many sufferers.

Of course, for those who experience cravings for sweet things in particular, the thought of cutting them out of their diet forever can be quite distressing. What some people have found helpful, therefore, is to eliminate sugar from their diets for a period of a month, during which time the cravings subside considerably, and then add it back in at a lower level.

The Good Stuff

Even if no particular food triggers can be identified, maintaining a healthier diet will provide long-term benefits to anyone who suffers from fibromyalgia or MPS. Eating the right types of foods will ensure that your body receives all the nutrients it requires and is able to absorb them effectively, and that toxins are eliminated efficiently.

Greater quantities of raw or lightly cooked fruits and vegetables, especially organic ones, should be introduced into the diet, and red meats which are high in fat should be replaced with fish or lean poultry. Polyunsaturated vegetable oils, meanwhile, should be replaced with extra virgin olive oil. Whole grains, too, are very good for the body, but of course if any of these foodstuffs appear to be contributing to your symptoms, then reduce your intake or remove them from your diet completely. If necessary, you can use vitamins and supplements to ensure that your body is getting everything that it needs.

Drinking plenty of fresh, still water is also essential for good health. Six to eight glasses (around 1.5 litres) per day is recommended to keep the body well hydrated and, as one of the benefits of drinking water is that it improves concentration, it is especially important that those with fibromyalgia have their daily intake.

As we saw in Chapter 25, many sufferers of fibromyalgia and MPS have been found to be deficient in magnesium and, although supplements can of course be taken, there are certain foodstuffs which are high in this essential element, including:

- Halibut
- Dry roasted almonds, cashews and peanuts
- Soybeans
- Spinach
- Cereals such as shredded wheat
- Oatmeal and wheat bran
- Baked potatoes
- Black-eyed peas and kidney beans
- Brown rice
- Lentils
- Avocados
- Plain yoghurt
- Bananas
- Raisins

As the majority of the population is believed to be deficient in omega-3 fatty acids, increasing your consumption of fish such as Pacific herring, sardines, trout, salmon, mackerel and fresh tuna, as well as of flax seeds, walnuts and canola oil is likely to be highly beneficial in terms of maintaining overall good health, and may well help towards alleviating fibromyalgia and MPS symptoms.

Vegan Diets

The issue of vegan diets, which contain no meat, dairy products or eggs, is a slightly controversial one in general. Although one clinical trial showed that female sufferers of fibromyalgia who were put on a diet consisting of raw foods such as fruits, vegetables, nuts, seeds, legumes and cereals, as well as several varieties of fermented foods, experienced a significant reduction in pain and depression symptoms in particular, there are those who believe that such a strict regime causes more harm than good.

When considering any changes to your diet, always consult with your doctor first.

29

Exercise

Exercise has been found by numerous studies to be one of the most effective ways of managing fibromyalgia and MPS. In fact, most consider it not just beneficial, but essential in terms of reducing pain and fatigue, preventing muscle wastage, avoiding weight gain and improving overall mental and physical well-being.

The trouble is, though, that sufferers of these conditions often find themselves in a Catch 22 situation. The pain, stiffness and fatigue can make exercise feel all but impossible, but even when they do make the effort, the symptoms seem to worsen temporarily. For those who do persevere and get into the habit of exercising regularly, however, the benefits have proved to make it well worthwhile.

Part of the reason why some patients have difficulty with exercise is because they try to do too much too soon. They either over-exert themselves or try to do exercises which are simply too difficult in the early days, and then become discouraged as a result. A far more effective approach, however, is to build up the levels of physical activity very gradually.

Stretching

Stretching is one of the most important parts of the exercise regime for fibromyalgia and MPS patients, both for the following reasons and as part of the warm-up for other types of activity. It:

- Helps to elongate the muscles and make them more elastic, which in turn reduces stiffness and pain
- Helps to relax tense muscles and prevent soreness
- Allows you to achieve greater range of motion by increasing your flexibility

- Helps to reduce muscle cramps
- May help you to get to sleep more quickly and enjoy sounder sleep
- Is a great way to relax

Stretching, though, is not just stretching, and there are, in fact, many different types of stretching exercises which can be carried out. Care does need to be taken, however, because some of these put too much stress on the muscles and joints, and it is therefore advisable that you take advice from your health care provider or physical therapist in order to avoid further pain or injury.

Whatever types of stretching exercise are recommended for you to do, here are a few tips to bear in mind:

- Even though stretching exercises can be used to warm up before other forms of activity, sufferers of fibromyalgia and MPS will need to warm up before stretching. A warm bath or shower or a quick walk around the house should help to get your muscles ready for action.
- Remember that the aim is not to go at your stretching exercises like a bull at a gate. Start with just a single repetition and then build up gradually to five or more.
- Focus on your breathing as you stretch. Breathe in deeply through your nose and then out through your mouth.
- Your stretches should only take you to the point where you can feel some resistance in your muscles, so never hold a stretch until it causes you pain.
- If a particular muscle feels especially painful, then do not push it. Either do fewer repetitions or hold the stretch for a shorter space of time.
- If you feel very stiff, then try stretching in warm water which will make it feel less painful.

Low Impact Aerobic Exercise

Low impact aerobic exercise such as walking or using a treadmill or an exercise bike can be very beneficial for fibromyalgia and MPS sufferers, but anything which puts undue amounts of pressure on the muscles or joints or jars the body, such as jogging and sports like basketball, should be avoided. Again though, as with stretching exercises, it is important to start slow with around five minutes' exercise every other day, gradually building up to 30–60 minutes four times per week.

Swimming

Many fibromyalgia and MPS patients find that swimming or water exercise is ideally suited to their condition because of course there is no weight or pressure on the muscles and joints. Swimming or exercising in a heated pool can be especially beneficial as the warm water helps to relax and soothe the muscles.

Whatever type of exercise regime you start on, try to be prepared for setbacks and do not let them make you feel discouraged. Perseverance really does pay off when it comes to exercise, so do try to stick with it. Also, do not forget that if one type of exercise seems to be having little effect, or if you are finding it hard to stick to, then you can always try something different. Many people, for example, find working on exercise machines quite boring, but are quite happy to exercise in water, so find what works for you and keep going.

Breathing Exercises

Aside from regular exercise, many people find that breathing exercises can also help to alleviate the muscle tension which leads to the pain of fibromyalgia and MPS. By practising breathing exercises for a few minutes every day, you can essentially retrain yourself to breathe more deeply at all times, introducing higher levels of oxygen into your bloodstream and relaxing muscle tension.

30

Posture

As we have already seen, either naturally poor posture, or that which results from an accident or injury, or from compensating for pain by holding certain parts of the body in unnatural ways, can not only do much to increase pain symptoms for those with fibromyalgia and MPS, but can even lead to the formation of new trigger points. In many cases, however, patients are not even aware that their posture is bad and so it is important that they be assessed by an expert.

Poor posture is actually one of the main culprits when it comes to neck and back pain in particular. Especially in cases where the individual spends long amounts of time slumped in a chair or in front of a computer, quite severe pain can result from the stress and tension which is placed on the muscles.

While a greater awareness of your posture is the essential first step to correcting it, there are also exercises which can be taught to help alleviate the situation. In addition, patients can learn about the principles of good posture and re-train themselves to walk, sit and lie in more healthy ways.

Of course, choosing the right types of chairs and mattresses is also an important part of improving posture, and ergonomically-designed furniture in the home and the workplace can play a big part in encouraging sufferers to sit correctly and so lessen their pain.

In more serious cases where poor posture is an issue, patients may even be recommended to wear a back brace to stabilise the spinal column or support muscles which have become especially fatigued.

31

Sleep and Fatigue

Aside from the terrible pain which is experienced by those with fibromyalgia and MPS, the chronic fatigue and sleeplessness is enough to drive many to despair. Unfortunately though, this is another area where a Catch 22 situation can very easily develop. The pain and discomfort makes sleep extremely difficult and then the symptoms are made even more severe by the lack of sleep and the stress associated with being constantly tired.

Of course, getting a good night's sleep is essential for everyone. Not only does it help us to feel refreshed and ready to face the day ahead, but it is also during the time when we are in the deepest stages of sleep that our bodies work on healing themselves. Sleep deprivation, even for one night, can leave us feeling grumpy, groggy, irritable and forgetful, as well as affecting our ability to concentrate and our attention spans. If it continues, the memory can become even more impaired and the part of the brain which controls language, planning and the sense of time is also affected. In one study, it was found that the symptoms of fibromyalgia could be reproduced, simply by depriving the individuals who took part of sleep.

There are, however, a number of things that fibromyalgia and MPS patients can do to try to improve their sleep patterns, and it is these that we are going to consider here.

Establish a healthy sleep regime
Going to bed and getting up at irregular hours is not conducive to achieving sound and restful sleep, so set yourself a regular time for both and stick to it, even at weekends and when you are on holiday.

Make your environment conducive to sleep

Make sure that your bed and bedroom are comfortable, that the room temperature is moderate and that there is plenty of ventilation. In addition, minimise any light coming into the room.

Although it is common nowadays for people to watch television in bed before trying to drop off to sleep, all this does is to keep the brain active and stop it from relaxing. Your bedroom should be reserved exclusively for sleep and sexual relations.

Avoid naps

Clearly, if you nap during the day, and especially during the afternoon or early evening, you are not going to feel tired enough to get off to sleep at night.

Avoid alcohol and caffeine before bedtime

Alcohol and caffeine are both strong stimulants and in order to get a really restful night's sleep, you need to avoid either for 4–6 hours before going to bed.

Avoid any fluids just before bedtime

Even drinks which do not contain any kind of stimulant can cause interruptions to your sleep if you find yourself having to get up and make treks to the toilet. So, no fluids at all just before bedtime.

Avoid large meals before bedtime

Eating a heavy meal and then going straight to bed means that your body is still trying to digest the food when it should be winding down for the night. Not only is sleep likely to be harder to come by, but there is every chance that you could wake up with indigestion or stomach ache.

Going to sleep on an empty stomach which is growling and complaining, however, is also not a good idea. If you feel hungry, therefore, just opt for a light snack.

Avoid exercise before bedtime

Although many people imagine that exercising just before going to bed would be conducive to a better night's sleep, in fact the opposite is true. The stimulation of the heart, brain and muscles, as well as the increase in body temperature, all make getting to sleep very much harder and so exercise should be avoided within the three hours before bedtime.

If sleep eludes you

If you get into bed and still find yourself unable to sleep after 15 or 20 minutes, then tossing and turning will only cause greater frustration. Instead, get up and go into a different room and read or do some other quiet activity. Only when you begin to feel sleepy should you go back to bed and try again.

Little and often

Where chronic fatigue is one of your symptoms, try to do little and often and try to time your activities so that things such as light house-work are done around mid-morning or whenever you feel at your best. Doing too much at any one time only aggravates fatigue symptoms, so try not to overdo it so that you feel inclined to nap during the day and spoil your night's sleep.

Medications

Although sleeping pills are generally best avoided, both because they can impair the quality of the deep sleep that we need and because many of these medications are highly addictive, your doctor may be able to prescribe a mild dose of a tricyclic antidepressant to help with sleep problems. If there is an underlying cause for your sleep distur-bances, such as sleep apnea, restless leg syndrome or teeth grinding, then it is important that your doctor identifies this so that he or she can advise accordingly.

32

Stress Management

As most sufferers of fibromyalgia and MPS will be highly aware, these are both conditions which are very sensitive to stress. Even slight amounts of stress can cause symptoms to worsen and severe flare-ups to occur, so the ability to manage it effectively can lead to a much improved quality of life.

Although of course the old adage that 'prevention is better than cure' applies equally to stress as to most other things, sometimes it is not entirely avoidable, so in this chapter I am going to suggest a number of ways to both avoid and reduce stress levels. Remember though, that you do not have to stick to using just one technique, and in fact many sufferers find that using a combination of methods is most effective.

Avoiding Stress

In order to be able to avoid stress, we first of all need to be aware of what our stress triggers are. In some cases, it might be certain people that get us going, whereas in others it could be situations or even substances. When we know which are the ones to set us off though, then we can do something about them.

Avoiding People

People can be at the root of a great deal of our stress, whether they mean to be or not. Some just seem to have an uncanny knack of pushing our buttons, while others can drive us to despair with their negativity, their gossiping or their inability to listen. Knowing which people you want to retain a relationship with and which ones are just increasing your stress levels and making your life more difficult can be key to avoiding stress.

Discovering that you are suffering from a chronic illness may not be the best way to find out who your friends are, but it is certainly an effective one. You may find that certain people who were probably only on the fringes of your life and not particularly supportive anyway, just simply seem to disappear. If this happens naturally, then let it, because the chances are that their lack of interest or support would only become intensely irritating and stressful in any case.

On the other hand, there will also be people who are quite prepared to stick around, but with whom you have difficult relationships. Ask yourself what these people add to your life and if the answer is 'nothing', then do what you can to limit your contact with them or wave them goodbye altogether. It might sound harsh, but you really do get to choose who you have in your life and you need to question how much they really care about you if they are not prepared to support you.

Avoiding Situations

There are, of course, numerous situations that we humans find stressful. Getting stuck in traffic jams, being in crowds, arguing with the people that we care about and being in debt all have the potential to raise our levels of anxiety, even when we are otherwise fit and healthy. With fibromyalgia and MPS, however, you may find that there are things that stress you which did not previously, such as being in places with bright lights or loud noises. Think about the situations when you can feel your stress levels soaring and then do your best to avoid them.

Avoiding Substances

As we discussed in Chapter 28, certain foods and drinks can play havoc with fibromyalgia and MPS symptoms, causing painful flare-ups which in turn increase stress levels. Try to identify which particular substances cause bad reactions and then eliminate them from your diet. In addition, if you find that being in a smoke-filled atmosphere or one with strong chemical smells is troublesome for you, then stay away.

Routine as an Avoidance Tactic

The unexpected and constantly being faced with life's ups and downs can be extremely stressful to many people, but evening out the bumps by getting yourself into a routine can make things much more manageable. While it might sound slightly boring, knowing what is around the corner can help enormously to alleviate feelings of stress and relieve the pressure to make instant decisions and react on the spur of the moment.

Planning and Scheduling

Planning and scheduling is, of course, part and parcel of developing a routine, but it also means that you will be able to avoid trying to do too much. Rushing around like a maniac to fit everything in is certain to raise stress levels, so schedule only a limited number of activities which allow for some of the 'must dos' and the 'nice to dos', but be sure to leave sufficient time in between so that there is no need to hurry.

Rest

Sometimes, when things feel like they are likely to start getting on top of us physically, mentally or emotionally, the best way to avoid stress is simply to take some rest. Planning a period of rest, and knowing that we have it to look forward to, can also be a great stress-buster.

Reducing Stress

As we have said, sometimes heading stress off at the pass simply is not an option and we find ourselves facing anxiety-provoking situations and events. What matters in these circumstances is not the situation or event itself though, but rather how we react to it and handle it. Here, therefore, is a range of suggestions of things that you can try to reduce your stress levels, and with them your pain and fatigue symptoms.

Physical Relaxation and Therapies

In Chapter 24, we looked at a number of different physical therapies, including different massage techniques and acupuncture, which many fibromyalgia and MPS sufferers find extremely helpful in terms of relieving the pain of their conditions. These therapies, however, also provide the benefit of physical relaxation and can be excellent ways to lower stress levels, as can a visit to a steam room, a long soak in the bath and even stretching exercises. Putting aside a minute or two to practice slow deep-breathing exercises can also make you feel instantly more relaxed, and of course this is something that you can do anywhere and at any time.

Meditation

The ancient art of meditation, if practiced regularly, can be particularly helpful in reducing stress levels and can easily be combined with periods of rest throughout the day. Meditation involves concentrating your mind so that it is free from distraction and you might, for example, concentrate on your breathing so that it fills your awareness to the exclusion of everything else around you. Slow meditative physical exercise such as tai chi can also be extremely beneficial for both body and mind.

Relaxation Tapes and Music Therapy

Listening to relaxation tapes is one of the most popular methods used for de-stressing, and recordings of everything from soothing music to jungle sounds and whale noises are easily available in the shops. Find which suits you best and then sit comfortably or lie down in a quiet room and soak up the relaxing atmosphere.

Of course, music tapes too can be great for relieving stress, but be careful which music you choose. Anything too loud, fast or angry-sounding will only serve to wind you up further and anything which has connections with bad experiences in the past will only make matters worse.

Time Out

In this fast-paced world where we seem to be constantly in the company of other people, it can be very easy to forget the simple pleasure of being alone. Whether you simply take time out to lie down in a relaxing and comfortable environment, sit down to read quietly or take a walk on your own, just being away from others can really help to clear your head, make you feel calmer and push stress to one side.

Facing Problems Head-On

Sometimes the things which cause us stress are ones which simply go round and round in our heads but never find any resolution. Rather than avoiding the issue or simply letting feelings of stress circulate in the background, try focusing on coming up with practical solutions and strategies which will solve the problem. While it is important not to let yourself become overwhelmed, if you take one thing at a time, you can gradually gnaw away at the things which are causing your stress and you might even come up with some truly inspirational ideas.

Do What You Enjoy

People who suffer from fibromyalgia and MPS typically live with huge amounts of guilt about all the things they feel they ought to be doing but cannot do. As a consequence, often they feel that they do not deserve to take time out for the things that they actually enjoy. In fact though, living a life which is filled with guilt, difficulties and drudgery, not to mention pain and fatigue, and not experiencing any fun and enjoyment, simply adds to the feelings of stress and will send you into a downward spiral.

No matter what our situation, we all need and deserve some enjoyment in life. How we get that enjoyment does not have to be through something earth-shattering or major, but can be from simple things such as playing a board game with the family, watching a favourite television show or spending an evening with friends. Never forget that it is not your fault that you are suffering from a chronic condition and that you deserve fun and enjoyment just as much as the next person. When your stress levels are lowered through fun activities, your life will feel much more manageable and you will likely feel capable of much more.

Using Humour

We have all heard the old saying 'Laughter is the best medicine', but remember that sayings such as this do not come from nowhere and in fact laughter really does help to reduce stress and pain, as well as to relieve conflicts. When we laugh, endorphins (the body's 'feel-good' hormones) are released, and these give us an overall sense of well-being and can even bring temporary relief from pain. Levels of stress hormones drop too and any physical tension leaves the body.

Whenever you feel as though stress is getting the better of you, reach for your favourite comedy programmes or films, or pick up the phone and relive some of those priceless funny moments that you have shared with friends or family.

Managing Expectations

Trying to live up to high or unrealistic expectations of ourselves and others is a sure fire way to create stress in life as all it does is lead to resentment, self-loathing and guilt. Trying to achieve perfection when you sometimes find it hard to imagine how you are even going to make it through the day is not realistic. If the housework has to wait, then let it wait, because in the greater scheme of things, what does it really matter?

Also, think about the expectations that you have of others. If you have your own ideas about what they 'should' be doing or saying, and how they 'should' be demonstrating their understanding and responding to your illness, then you are likely to feel disappointment and even resentment. The fact is that we are all different and the people who care about you will have their own ways of showing it, so let them do it in their own way and be grateful for it and you are much more likely to keep your stress levels under control.

Adjusting Your Thinking

We all have those little negative voices in our heads that eat away at our sense of optimism and self-confidence, and when you are suffering from a chronic illness such as fibromyalgia or MPS, these little voices can often take over, causing huge amounts of stress. They tell you that you are not doing well enough or that you will never be well again and can send you into a pit of despair. They can, however, be silenced, and all it takes is to talk back to them. Whenever you catch yourself thinking negative thoughts, turn them around to something positive, such as 'I am good enough' or 'I am doing so much better'. Instead of thinking 'I am sick and tired of feeling sick and tired', think 'I have the absolute freedom and power to change how I respond to any situation at any time'.

Another way in which it is important to adjust your thinking is by considering what is and is not your problem or responsibility. As we know, the vast majority of people who suffer from fibromyalgia and MPS are women, and women in particular can feel inclined to take care of others and, in some cases, to accept responsibility for them and their problems. When you find yourself feeling stressed about a situation, really stop and ask yourself whether it is your problem or responsibility or somebody else's. If it is the former, then break down the problem and deal with it bit by bit. If it genuinely belongs to someone else though, then step back and let that person deal with it themselves. Do not consider this a selfish act, but remember that you have your own concerns to deal with (and your own stress to contend with) and that stepping in to bail others out only robs them of the opportunity to learn for themselves.

Creative Activities

As I have already said, it is important to take time out for fun and pleasurable activities such as playing games, taking weekend breaks and even just watching your favourite television programme. In addition to this, however, creative pursuits in particular have several vital roles to play.

No matter whether drawing, painting, needlework, calligraphy, card-making or stamp collecting appeals to you, these are all hobbies which are quiet and peaceful, which help with your concentration and which provide a great deal of personal satisfaction. Immersing yourself in activities such as these can transport you to a place of pleasure which is a million miles away from all of your stressful thoughts and feelings, so find out where your passions lie and let your hobbies do just that.

Writing

Writing, even if it is done purely for our own benefit, is an activity which many people find extremely cathartic. All too often, the things that are causing us stress just go round and round in our heads and we can find no sense of relief. The simple act of getting our thoughts and feelings out and on paper, however, not only helps us to let go of them, but in many cases also helps us to find solutions which were not previously apparent.

Try keeping a stress journal in which you can let all of those demons free. Write about your deepest, darkest fears, let out your feelings of anger, disappointment, guilt or shame and remember that this is for nobody else's eyes other than your own so you can afford to let rip. Just getting the feelings out will make you feel as though a huge weight has been lifted from your shoulders.

Being Assertive

Again, it is an unfortunate fact that far more women suffer from fibromyalgia and MPS than men, and generally speaking women tend to have greater problems with assertiveness than do their male counterparts. Being more assertive when you can no longer do all the things that you used to do is a vital skill to learn. You might always have said 'Yes' to everything in the past, for whatever reasons, but doing so now will only make your life unmanageable and highly stressful. While there is, of course, absolutely nothing wrong in letting those closest to you and who are most supportive of you know that they can count on you whenever you are able, investing time and effort in those who give nothing in return will cause your stress levels to rocket.

Although many women tend to think of saying 'No' as being selfish and uncaring, setting reasonable limits and boundaries is healthy. You may well have certain responsibilities to others, but you also have responsibilities to yourself, and one of those is to ensure that your physical and mental health is taken care of.

Asking for Help

There will almost inevitably be times when you simply feel unable to deal with the things that are causing you stress, even if this is just tackling a backlog of housework. If this is the case, then reach out to the people around you and ask for their support instead of letting it worry you half to death.

Asking for help is not always easy for many people, but an important thing to remember here is that the people who care for you probably feel helpless in many ways and would gladly give of their time and energy to do something which genuinely makes a difference to your life. If you do not allow them this opportunity on occasions and insist on being totally self-reliant, not only will they feel shut out, but your stress levels will continue to climb into the bargain.

Medications

Should you find that you are becoming overwhelmed by stress and that nothing else seems to provide relief, then there is, of course, medication which can help. Antidepressant drugs such as the selective serotonin reuptake inhibitor (SSRI) Zoloft can be very effective at treating panic, anxiety and depression and, while many people prefer to avoid taking medications such as these, ultimately if you are finding it difficult to cope otherwise, the benefits may well outweigh the drawbacks.

Dealing with Major Life Events and Crises

While some major life events can be planned for in advance so that any stress or disruption is kept to a minimum, of course others arrive out of the blue and take us totally by surprise. Ironically, even what should be some of the most pleasurable moments of our lives, such as getting married, moving to a wonderful new home or seeing our first grandchild into the world can still be incredibly stressful, let alone the intensely painful ones which come when we perhaps lose someone close to us unexpectedly.

In the case of those major life events which are planned or expected, you can of course use any of the strategies that we have just outlined to help see you through. It is still important to remember, however, that even if something is expected, we do not always react as we imagined we would. We may, for example, think that we are prepared for the loss of a loved one after a long illness, but when it actually happens we can feel totally hijacked by our feelings and emotions in a way which leaves us feeling shocked and bewildered.

Probably one of the most valuable things to remember when faced with major situations and crises is a little thing called the Serenity Prayer, the mantra of those in 12-step programmes such as Alcoholics Anonymous.

God grant me the serenity
to accept the things I cannot change;

courage to change the things I can;
and wisdom to know the difference.

You do not have to be a recovering alcoholic or even a believer in God for these few simple lines to be able to offer immense comfort, because all they really do is help to put things into perspective. Truly understanding and appreciating where you have real power in your life can make handling highly stressful situations and events much more manageable.

Another thing which is worth bearing in mind is the fact that nothing, and I mean absolutely nothing in life lasts forever. However hard that might be to imagine when you are in the depths of despair and feel like you have hit rock bottom, it is literally true for everything, so try hard not to let yourself become overwhelmed because the situation will change.

On a more practical note, there are few if any of us who can get through really tough situations and crises without some kind of external help, and it is important to seek out as many positive sources of support as you can find. The bigger the crisis, the more support you are likely to need, but that is perfectly okay – just keep talking. Whether you turn to family members, friends, your local church, doctors, psychologists, lawyers or whoever will, of course, be determined by the circumstances, but whoever you happen to need, call on them and do not try to cope with the situation yourself.

Taking good care of yourself, while it might be the last thing on your mind when you are in the midst of a crisis, is actually more important than ever. If you begin to get stressed, start to overdo things or skip your periods of rest, you will be less well equipped to cope with the situation either mentally or physically. Letting these things slide will only add to your problems rather than alleviating them.

Be patient and forgiving of yourself in the face of major life events and crises and never forget that any choices or decisions you make are the best ones that you are capable of making. Also, remember that there is no right or wrong in terms of your feelings and there is no deadline on how long you are 'supposed' to feel a certain way. If you do feel that you have become stuck, however, and the feelings remain intense and show no sign of lifting, then do seek help from your doctor. Use a diary to write down your feelings and in this way you are likely to accept them more readily and will be able to move on from them more quickly.

Dealing with major events in our lives has a nasty habit of uncovering all kinds of past hurts and difficulties that we thought had long since been laid to rest. If you feel that this is the case, then seek help from a professional therapist or counsellor who can help you to work through these.

33

How to Beat Brain Fog

Brain fog, or 'fibro fog' as it is commonly known, can in some ways have a more devastating effect on fibromyalgia sufferers than either the excruciating pain or the chronic fatigue. While the latter might be extremely hard to cope with, at least they do not directly involve anyone else.

When patients of fibromyalgia suffer from the dreaded fibro fog, their most common experience is of:

- Not being able to find the right words, coming out with entirely the wrong words and not being able to string a coherent sentence together
- Words coming out in a different order than when they were still inside the brain
- Not being able to form the words verbally which are inside the brain
- Losing their train of thought and just stopping mid-sentence
- Jumbled thoughts
- Not being able to spell words
- Forgetting things that have only just happened
- Forgetting things that you have only recently been told
- Forgetting people's names – even those of best friends
- Feelings of disorientation and forgetting where they are
- Feelings of detachment
- Not being able to concentrate and having a short attention span
- Not being able to read things properly
- Not being able to follow what is happening on the television
- Repeating things that they have already said – such as telling the same joke or story over and over again

When fibro fog attacks, it leaves its victims feeling stupid and self-conscious and it eats away at their confidence and seriously makes them wonder whether they are losing their intelligence. Frequently, this leads to feelings of agitation and then panic, which only add to the problem.

In some cases, fibromyalgia sufferers even get to the stage where they begin to avoid company and isolate themselves so as not to have to face the embarrassment that they feel. They might start to live their lives in the online environment where they have the safety of knowing that they can correct their jumbled sentences without anyone being the wiser. In others it can have a devastating effect on relationships with other people – imagine going on a third or fourth date and not being able to remember anything that your partner told you about him or herself previously or, worse still, confusing his or her details with somebody else's! Even friends can see you as being rude or disinterested when you cannot recall earlier conversations, however important they might have been.

What Makes Brain Fog Worse?

In most people's experience, there are certain things which make brain fog feel worse. Typically, these are:

- Constant interruptions in the conversation – regardless of whether it is themselves or someone else who is talking
- Conversations which go back and forth and have lots of interaction
- Loud voices or laughter
- Becoming flustered about getting things wrong and then focusing on the reactions of other people
- Conversations which go off at a tangent or get side-tracked

Unfortunately, when brain fog starts to descend and things start to come out all wrong in a conversation, the ensuing embarrassment and panic leads them into yet another Catch 22 situation in which the level of confusion just increases.

What Can You Do?

Cutting yourself off from the rest of the world is clearly not an ideal way to deal with fibro fog, but there are different methods which sufferers have discovered for themselves that do help.

Write things down – Keep notepads everywhere, at home, in the car, at the office and in your handbag or, if your brain fog gets so bad that you are unlikely to remember where you put the notebooks, write things in a diary that you take with you everywhere. Not only will your notes serve to remind you of things that you have forgotten, but the act of writing them in the first place will ensure that they are more deeply embedded in your mind.

Keep your mind active – Make a point of doing activities which keep your brain active and sharp, such as doing word or number puzzles or reading.

Keep your body active – Even moderate amounts of gentle exercise can help to clear your brain, as well as increasing your energy levels and helping with pain symptoms.

Break tasks up into manageable chunks – Taking on too much at once or trying to deal with a complex set of problems is only likely to lead to more confusion, so break your tasks up and deal with only one distinct part at a time.

Avoid distractions – If you are trying to concentrate on something or remember something, then make sure that you take yourself as far away as possible from where other people are talking, from where there is a television or radio playing or from where there is any other kind of distraction.

Move on – If you find yourself having lost your train of thought, just say 'I'm sorry, I can't remember what I was saying' and then wait for the other person to begin talking again. Also, remember that people who do not have fibromyalgia also have their 'senior moments' when they lose their thread, so try not to take it too much to heart.

Think before you speak – Depending upon how thick the fog is, this may or may not work, but some people have found that formulating what they want to say before trying to speak helps in certain circumstances.

Don't be afraid of silence – Many people feel uncomfortable with gaps and silences in conversations and will try to fill them, but if you find that you are getting lost in a sentence, then just stop, take a breath and formulate what you want to say, or find another way to phrase it. Some people even find it useful to forewarn the person they are talking to that, as one put it so nicely, 'There is a pile up on the highway between brain and mouth', by saying 'One second' before trying again.

Ask for a recap – Especially if you are around friends or family or anyone else who knows of your condition, if you cannot remember what they are talking about, then just ask one member of the party to give you a discreet recap of what has been discussed. Although I have come across people who pretend that they can remember what other people are talking about and simply nod and go along with the conversation, this can be a rather dangerous tactic, especially if you happen to come out with a completely different viewpoint or opinion than you expressed previously.

Make sure that you address your other symptoms – Lack of sleep, depression and being in pain all have effects on the brain which are likely to increase the incidence or severity of fibro fog, so be sure to seek out appropriate treatment for these other symptoms.

Manage your stress – Again, when you feel stressed and anxious, fibro fog is likely to be worse, so use the tips and suggestions in the previous chapter to keep your stress levels under control.

Lecithin – Lecithin is a substance which is found naturally in egg yolks, as well as in many plant and animal cells (including the cells of the human body), and is essential for the metabolism of fats. Some fibromyalgia patients have found that taking a supplement of lecithin has produced remarkable results in terms of improving the symptoms of fibro fog and fatigue.

How Can Other People Help?

Once you explain to those closest to you what it feels like to experience fibro fog, they will almost certainly want to do anything they can to help you through what might otherwise be very difficult conversations and interactions. Here are just a few things that they can do:

- Many of those who suffer from fibro fog find it far easier to keep track of a conversation when people speak to them at a normal volume or even fairly softly, so friends and family can help by keeping it down a little.

- Because looks of surprise, disbelief or amusement are likely to make the sufferer feel even more flustered and embarrassed, try to let any long pauses in the conversation or wrong words pass without comment.

- If the sufferer seems to have become lost in the conversation, either because he or she has forgotten what they were saying or because they cannot remember what was just said, discreetly put him or her back on track.

- If you are trying to have a conversation at a party or somewhere else where there is lots of noise and many distractions, find somewhere quieter to sit and talk.

34

Dealing with Irritable Bowel Syndrome

Irritable bowel syndrome (IBS), which is basically a problem with the functioning of the gut, including the bowels, frequently overlaps with fibromyalgia and MPS and, like these two conditions the cause of IBS is not clear and there is no known cure. Although all parts of the gut appear normal, even when examined microscopically, the condition can cause great discomfort due to abdominal pain and bloating, diarrhoea, constipation and nausea, which can in turn lead to feeling physically weak, an inability to eat and depression. The symptoms can change from day to day and, in some cases, those with the condition experience short-term bouts of the illness, whilst others live with it on a longer-term basis.

It is estimated that as many as 70% of fibromyalgia sufferers also have IBS and, where IBS co-exists with this or MPS, the symptoms of both conditions tend to be worse than for those who only have one of the illnesses on its own. Pain and chronic fatigue are exacerbated by IBS, and the severity and the frequency of IBS symptoms are made worse by fibromyalgia and MPS.

Despite being incurable, as with fibromyalgia and MPS, there are things that sufferers of IBS can do to help relieve their symptoms and ultimately to help stop the interplay between the illnesses.

Diet

Adjusting diet is a very useful form of self-help which many IBS sufferers find provides them with considerable relief, but alongside this, you should also look at your patterns of eating. Skipping meals and eating on the go, for example, can not only trigger or exacerbate IBS symptoms, but it can also lead to other illnesses affecting the gut and the digestive systems.

In the same way as for the main symptoms of fibromyalgia and MPS, keeping a record of what you eat and any IBS symptoms which appear to flare up afterwards will give you some useful clues as to which foods you are particularly sensitive to and need to avoid. Simply try cutting out the suspect foods from your diet and then reintroducing them one by one to see whether you experience any change in your symptoms. Watch out in particular for dairy products, products containing gluten and red meats.

One thing which is particularly worth noting in terms of IBS is the role of fibre or roughage in the diet. High amounts of fibre are found in foodstuffs such as fruit, vegetables, wholemeal bread and cereals and fibre is the part of the food which is not absorbed into the body and so needs to be excreted. Although many doctors recommend a diet which is high in fibre for those suffering from the symptoms of IBS, and in particular constipation, some studies have shown that this can actually make matters worse in some cases. As was described in Chapter 28, different foods and drinks affect different people in different ways, so when making any adjustments to diet, it is probably safer to ignore any wholesale suggestions with respect to trigger foods and concentrate solely on what works and does not work for you personally.

Another thing which is well worth considering is probiotics. Probiotics, which can be taken as a supplement in capsule or drink form and even in the form of particular probiotic food products such as cheese, yoghurt and ice cream, contain 'good' bacteria. These good bacteria help to ward off the bad bacteria in the gut and increasing their levels in the body can contribute to alleviating IBS symptoms. You can find probiotic products in chemists, but there is also usually a good range available nowadays in supermarkets.

Here are some useful tips to remember when considering your diet and eating patterns:

- Be sure to eat regularly.
- Sit down to eat and do not rush your mealtimes.
- As the caffeine in both tea and coffee can sometimes be a factor in

IBS, limit yourself to three cups per day or cut them out of your diet altogether if you identify them as causing worsened symptoms.

■ Drink 1.5 litres, or around 6–8 tumbler-sized glasses of still water every day as this will help to soften stools.

■ Keep carbonated drinks to a minimum.

■ Cut down on, or cut out completely, alcohol and smoking as these can also contribute to symptoms.

■ Check out the effect of fibre in your diet and either increase or decrease as appropriate.

■ Some artificial sweeteners which are added to sugar-free, diabetic and slimming products can cause problems, so avoid these if possible.

■ Oats and linseed are both very good for reducing wind and bloating.

Stress

As we know, heightened levels of stress and anxiety can affect the symptoms of fibromyalgia and MPS quite severely, and it can have the same effect in terms of those associated with IBS too, because of the messages sent between the brain and the gut. Working on improving your sleep patterns so that you get the proper amount of restorative sleep, minimising sources of stress and seeking counselling for any tough emotional difficulties can do much to provide relief.

Exercise

Taking regular but gentle exercise not only helps to keep the body functioning at optimum levels, but also contributes to a reduction in stress levels. Be sure to schedule in short periods of exercise every day.

Medication

Sometimes, adjusting your diet, cutting out stress and taking regular exercise on their own may not be enough to relieve the symptoms of IBS, in which case you might need to speak to your doctor about the possibility of using over-the-counter or prescription medication. While laxatives and stool softeners can be highly effective at treating constipation, medications such as Imodium work particularly well for diarrhoea. At the same time as slowing down the action of the bowel, they also help to reduce the abdominal pain and cramps which typically go along with diarrhoea.

Antispasmodic medicines, which can be taken on an 'as required' basis, are another option for those who suffer with spasm-type pains, and these work by relaxing the muscles in the wall of the gut. As there are several different types of antispasmodic, if one particular type does not appear to have much effect, it is always worth trying another, but whatever symptoms of IBS you are experiencing, always be sure to discuss these and any possible courses of treatment with your doctor.

Tricyclic antidepressants are also sometimes used to treat the symptoms of IBS, as well, of course, as those associated with fibromyalgia and myofascial pain themselves. Generally they would only be prescribed if the IBS symptoms were quite severe and ongoing and, unlike antispasmodic medicines, they would need to be taken regularly to have any beneficial effect.

35

Keeping a Journal

During the course of this book, we have mentioned on several occasions the value of keeping journals to record different types of food and drink and different activities which appear to trigger or aggravate symptoms. A stress journal is also a great way to identify the root causes of any mental or emotional distress and to help release any difficult feelings.

Another type of journal which it is well worthwhile keeping is, of course, a straightforward journal of your symptoms. This can be a particularly useful thing to take with you when you visit your doctor or pain management specialist, especially as it can be difficult to remember symptoms when they change so radically from one day to the next as is typically the case with fibromyalgia and MPS. If there are particular symptoms such as numbness which are causing you problems, then write down what you were doing prior to the onset and what you were doing when the symptom flared up to try and identify whether there is a specific trigger which you can avoid in the future.

Most of the journals that we have mentioned so far have been quite practical ones which are designed to help you to improve your immediate quality of life by addressing symptoms. People who are suffering from fibromyalgia and MPS can, however, find themselves focusing so hard on getting through each day that they either forget about the future or view it as something very dark and bleak. Keeping other types of journals which record those things which are important and relevant to your future, therefore, can really help you to see it as something full of brightness, promise and hope and so contribute to your mental, emotional and spiritual well-being.

One type of journal which will not only help to frame your future, but also to encourage you to take action in terms of moving on in your life with your condition is one in which you record your life goals. Start by thinking about all the things you want to do and then break each goal down into manageable steps that you can work towards on a daily basis. Being able to see that you are inching closer to them is incredibly motivating and will help to inspire a 'can do' attitude towards your life.

You might also like to think about keeping a journal in which you identify the good things in your life and the improvements and growth that you are making in order to focus on the positives rather than the negatives. A journal which is used to re-evaluate your beliefs and your behaviours, meanwhile, can help to provide a whole new perspective, not just on your illness, but also on your life in general. Just what are the things which are holding you back and how can you change your thoughts and behaviours to live a much more fulfilling life?

If relationships have been, or have become difficult for you, then you might choose to keep a journal which helps you to improve these. You might choose to write about your communication with others or about how you communicate effectively with yourself, but ultimately anything which helps you to understand yourself and those closest to you better will be of benefit.

Whatever type of journal you decide is most suitable for you, do not be afraid to really open up and explore your deepest thoughts, feelings, hopes and dreams, because only by doing this will you be able to make effective change in your life. Remember, it is for your eyes only, so do not worry about things sounding unrealistic or foolish.

Part Five

Special Considerations

36

Work Issues

One of the huge concerns that many people who are diagnosed with fibromyalgia or MPS have is how their work will be affected. Although most of the sufferers of these two conditions are women, nowadays of course, women contribute significantly in a financial sense to the household and in some cases they are the chief bread-winner. The prospect of trying to keep a job when some days see you feeling unable to even get out of bed can be a terrifying and depressing thought. You are not, however, without options, and in this chapter we are going to consider some of these, as well as looking at a few of your rights and some of the things that you can do to make your work life easier.

Continuing in Your Existing Job

Having possibly worked for many years to get where you are, the thought of having to change jobs because of your illness may not be a particularly palatable one, especially if you are doing something that you really enjoy. If you do not want to move on to find something less taxing though, then consider some of the following suggestions.

Flexible Work Patterns

Although in the past employees have been expected to work set hours from set locations, modern technology has done much to change work patterns in recent years. Increasingly, employers are open to their staff working flexible hours and quite often they are prepared to let employees work from home. In fact, home working affords many financial benefits for employers in a whole range of different fields as it helps them to cut down on accommodation, lighting and heating costs, for example.

Even for those employees who are in perfect health, working from home, on the odd occasion if not all or most of the time, can lead to far greater productivity. Without all the distractions which typically exist in an office environment, home workers often find that they not only do better work, but they get through it quicker.

Of course, for those who suffer from fibromyalgia or MPS, not having to travel backwards and forwards to work, being able to start later on in the day when perhaps symptoms are less severe, being able to arrange their work areas in such a way that they can work more comfortably (such as in an environment where there are no bright lights, temperature extremes, excessive noise, strong smells and so on) and being able to take regular breaks and get up to move around when required can make a huge difference to their quality of life and their output. If you are struggling in your current work environment, therefore, and think that such an arrangement might help, then do not be afraid to ask. After all, the very worst that can happen is that your boss says 'No'. Even if working from home turns out not to be a viable option, working flexible hours in itself could improve your situation immensely, as could cutting down to part-time hours or job sharing.

If you are currently involved in shift work and the effect on your sleeping patterns is very detrimental to your condition, then it may be worthwhile asking if you can be reassigned to different duties with more regular working hours, rather than putting your job at risk by having to take large amounts of time off.

Adaptations at Work

Employers are expected to make reasonable accommodation for their workers and in the case of those who are suffering from fibromyalgia or MPS, there are a few relatively inexpensive solutions which can greatly help to minimise discomfort and consequently improve productivity. Many organisations today have health and safety representatives who are available to do a workstation evaluation, so find out whether this is the case in your company and take advantage of the opportunity to ensure that your work space meets your needs.

Finding an ergonomically designed chair which provides good support is one of the most effective ways to help reduce the pain of fibromyalgia and MPS. Make sure that if the chair has arms, these are adjustable, so that you can sit at the right distance from the desk and from the computer screen, if you use one. The height of the chair should also be adjustable so that when using a keyboard your arms are parallel to your thighs, and your screen should sit at eye level. Arm supports and wrist rests are also a cheap but effective way to reduce strain.

Small items of equipment such as copy holders and telephone headsets can also be very helpful, and if your job involves a great deal of typing and mouse clicking, then speech recognition software could also be a wise investment.

If your work area is particularly noisy, leaves you subjected to extremes of temperature or particular smells which upset you, or is too brightly lit, then find out whether there is a more suitable area that you could move to. In addition, try to ensure that your desk is located close to the facilities that you use most often.

Whatever adaptations are made to your work area, however, do remember to take regular breaks to get up and move around, as this will help to reduce the risk of repetitive strain injuries which can contribute to the formation of increased numbers of tender or trigger points.

Another thing that you might find useful is to arrange parking close to your workplace so that you can avoid long walks. If your company has its own car park, perhaps you could have a closer spot reserved for you.

Stress

While most jobs involve some amount of stress, for fibromyalgia and MPS sufferers it is important that this be minimised. Try to avoid stressful situations if at all possible and also try to find somewhere quiet where you can rest and do some relaxation exercises during rest and lunch breaks.

Coping with Brain Fog

Coping with brain fog or fibro fog can be enough of a challenge in your personal and social life, but trying to cope with it in the workplace can leave you and others wondering whether you are still up to the job. Getting written instructions for your work tasks and help in prioritising your assignments can help immensely in ensuring that nothing gets missed. Using memory aids such as organisers, diaries and wall planners and comprehensive electronic to-do lists which flag up reminders will all help to jog your memory and, especially if you deal with people outside your own organisation, contact management software which is completed with lots of detail will save you from the embarrassment of forgetting or confusing people's details.

Again, if your work area is noisy, find out if there is somewhere else that you could move to on a permanent basis, or even just ask for permission to use a quiet meeting room when you need to concentrate and the fibro fog has descended.

Sick Leave

Many companies specify their arrangements in relation to sick leave in their work contracts, outlining how many days of sick leave you are entitled to and precisely what will happen if you exceed the maximum. Make sure that you are familiar with these so that you do not get any nasty shocks further on down the road.

The other thing to remember about taking time off sick when you suffer from a condition which has no visible symptoms and is very poorly understood is that your manager and the people in your HR department may need some education if they are to believe that any time taken from work is justified. Find out whether your health care provider has any fact sheets about the illness or print off some information from the internet to fill any gaps in their knowledge. Also, be sure to follow the company's policies and procedures in terms of notifying them that you will not be going to work and providing them with self-certificated sick forms or sick notes from your doctor.

Changing Jobs

If your current job requires a great deal of physical exertion or has otherwise become too taxing or stressful for you to manage, then you can of course consider changing jobs and finding something less demanding. What many people fear in this situation, however, is that the very fact that they have fibromyalgia or MPS will immediately cause them to be rejected as a candidate.

Health-Related Questions

As I mentioned a few moments ago, employers are expected to make reasonable provisions for workers who are sick or disabled, and in addition they are limited as to what they can ask you at a job interview. Their questions should be focused on establishing whether you have the required skills and abilities to do the job; and they are not allowed to ask you outright whether you have any physical or mental disabilities, although they can ask whether there is anything that would stop you from being able to fulfil the role given reasonable accommodation if required. Only with your express consent can they approach your doctor for your medical records.

Reasonable Accommodation

Asking a prospective employer to make reasonable accommodation for your condition should not, by law, count you out of the running, but remember the word 'reasonable'. Trying to justify a request for the great big plush office at the corner of the building because the lighting is better may be a tad tricky, but asking for a chair and other pieces of equipment to suit your needs is certainly not unreasonable.

As an aside here, if you do decide to look for alternative employment, bear in mind that working outdoors could be very challenging, especially if you suffer from sensitivity to extremes of temperature or changes in temperature.

Self-Employment

For some people with fibromyalgia or MPS, working from home on a self-employed basis not only gets around the workplace issues quite nicely, but even allows them to fulfil what may have been a long-held dream. Working the number of hours to suit themselves and determining their own start and finish times can make life considerably easier, but it is also important to remember that being self-employed can be highly stressful, and stress of course can make the symptoms of these conditions very much worse.

If you are going to consider self-employment, then be realistic and really do your homework. Even if you just want to set up a low-cost service business, you will still need some money behind you to see you through the period when you are finding clients and building your business up. Being self-employed can also be very lonely, so if your illness is already making you feel quite isolated, self-employment may not be for you.

Giving Up Work Altogether

Of course, most of us need to work for a living in order to keep the wolf from the door, but if your financial situation allows, you may consider giving up work altogether. Really give this some careful consideration though, because even if you think you could manage comfortably in terms of money, there is still the potential for stress to be created by the loss of self-esteem.

37

Disability

For those sufferers of fibromyalgia or MPS who find it impossible to continue working and earning, there is the option of claiming disability and any financial benefits associated with this. Although making a case for disability if you have either of these two conditions, however, is not always easy and for several reasons.

In order to claim the care and mobility components of Disability Living Allowance in the UK, an individual must prove two things beyond any reasonable doubt. The first of these is that you actually suffer from the condition, and the second is that it makes your life difficult, if not intolerable. To claim the care component, clearly you need to demonstrate that you do actually need care as a result of your condition too. Because so little is generally understood about fibromyalgia and MPS, as well as other illnesses such as myalgic encephalomyelitis (ME) and chronic fatigue syndrome, coming up with a firm diagnosis can be extremely difficult and some doctors take a considerable amount of time to rule out all other possibilities. If this is a route that you want to take, therefore, then you need to ensure that you deal with a specialist in the illnesses who can help you to build a stronger case.

Because there are no visible internal or external signs for doctors to go on, patients who wish to claim disability have no choice other than to cite their pain as the major cause. Pain, however, is a purely subjective sensation; indeed many people suffer persistent pain without being disabled, all of which means that many doctors are reluctant to declare patients of fibromyalgia and MPS as disabled. In addition, of course, there are still physicians who insist that fibromyalgia and MPS are psychological rather than physical illnesses and that the pain is all in the patients' heads.

Another thing which often makes doctors reluctant to declare patients with these conditions as disabled is that the extent to which they are able to live a 'normal' life is affected by how each individual copes with the symptoms and the extent to which they accept their condition. Whilst two people with fibromyalgia, for example, might suffer the same levels of absolute pain, one might accept the diagnosis, take all the recommended steps to improve their situation and consequently be able to cope quite well, whereas the other might live in denial, do nothing and sink into anxiety and depression and, effectively, into disability.

Even if a sufferer's own doctor has reached a diagnosis of fibromyalgia or MPS, an application for financial benefits may lead to a requirement for them to face yet another battery of tests and a separate diagnosis from an independent physician or consultant. In some cases, patients have been known to have waited up to two years for the initial diagnosis, let alone face a second one. Having said this, however, there is a general consensus that every case should be thoughtfully evaluated according to the individual's own unique set of circumstances, and so if your condition has led to you requiring care or your mobility is so badly affected that your life has become difficult or intolerable, then the option does exist for you to make a claim for the relevant financial allowance.

38

Pregnancy

Pregnancy can raise two key issues in relation to fibromyalgia and MPS. First of all, some women only experience the first symptoms of their condition during pregnancy, which leads to even greater problems with diagnosis, and secondly, the symptoms of these illnesses are frequently exacerbated by being pregnant.

Pregnancy can be a tiring business, even in cases where the mother is in perfect health and, of course, it can be the bearer of muscle stiffness and pain. This means that there is the potential for doctors to misdiagnose the symptoms of fibromyalgia and MPS as normal pregnancy symptoms. It also means that pregnant women who suffer from either of these conditions can effectively be hit with a 'double whammy'.

Several studies have shown that pregnant women experienced a worsening of fibromyalgia and MPS symptoms, with greater levels of pain, stiffness and fatigue being reported by as many as 80% of sufferers. The third trimester was the period when the greatest deterioration occurred and the increase in the severity of symptoms often continued for around three months after delivery. In addition, women with these conditions appeared to be more vulnerable to postnatal depression than those without. Thankfully, however, there was no indication that having either fibromyalgia or MPS has any effect on the baby, which has just the same chances of being born at full term and at a normal weight.

Interestingly though, and despite the findings of these studies, anecdotal evidence seems to suggest that for some women, pregnancy actually brings about an improvement in their symptoms. Once the period of morning sickness is over, expectant mothers often begin to feel much better and overall they do very well during pregnancy.

Preparing for Pregnancy

Any woman, regardless of her state of health, is recommended to take steps to prepare her body for pregnancy, both to ensure that conception takes place more easily and so that her body is properly equipped to carry the baby safely throughout the full term. General recommendations include:

- Stopping smoking
- Avoiding alcohol
- Stopping all non-essential medicines and drugs
- Avoiding X-rays, including dental X-rays
- Avoiding soft, unpasteurised and blue cheeses, uncooked eggs, peanuts and liver, as well as products containing liver such as paté
- Cutting down on caffeine
- Taking essential vitamins and minerals
- Taking folic acid to help with the formation of the foetus

In addition, a diet which includes the following is suggested for at least three months before the planned conception:

- Fresh fruits and vegetables
- Peas, beans and lentils
- Seeds and nuts
- Oily fish
- Organic dairy products
- Lean fresh meat

Ensuring that levels of vitamin B and magnesium are sufficient is vital in the run-up to pregnancy. Vitamin B is necessary to help with the ripening of the egg before conception and magnesium is required to build healthy cell membranes.

Another important aspect of ensuring optimum health at the pre-conception stage is, of course, exercise. For sufferers of fibromyalgia or MPS, however, it is important that in their efforts to prepare themselves they do not push themselves too far or to the point where they suffer flare-ups. Also, they are advised to wait until they are not in a flare before trying to conceive. As at all times, they should do whatever possible to avoid stress.

Breastfeeding

Most doctors would recommend that babies be breast fed, at least for the first few vital months of their lives, but while doing so does have the advantage to fibromyalgia and MPS sufferers of carrying less weight, the prolonged periods of time spent feeding can cause them to become stiff and sore. It is important, therefore, to ensure that you have good support for your arms, legs and back while feeding, or you could try placing your baby in a sling to support its weight or feed whilst lying down.

Because stress can not only cause painful flare-ups in symptoms but also interrupt the 'let down' reflex, nursing mums should try to make their environments as relaxing as possible. Ensure that the room is warm, comfortable and private and, if it helps you to relax, try playing some soothing music while you are feeding.

Taking Medications

Medications can pass into the bloodstream of the unborn child through the mother's breast milk. As many of the drugs which are used to treat fibromyalgia and MPS are not suitable for use during pregnancy and breastfeeding, it is important to discuss any plans for pregnancy with your doctor beforehand. If you are taking any medications for your condition and the pregnancy is unplanned, however, do not discontinue their use, but do talk to your doctor at the very earliest opportunity. Remember too, that some herbal treatments can also be dangerous for pregnant and nursing mothers, so again, check with your doctor to ensure that anything you are taking is safe.

In some cases, women who suffer from fibromyalgia or MPS have to return to drug treatment in order to control their symptoms after the birth and so are unable to continue breastfeeding. While this might be disappointing, it is important to remember that it only takes a very short period of time for babies to get the benefit of their mother's immune system and that bottle feeding does provide the advantage that others can help with the feeding routine.

Precautions

While massage, gentle exercise and stretching, both in and out of water can be beneficial in terms of easing the symptoms of fibro-myalgia and MPS during pregnancy, do avoid very hot baths, heat pads and electric blankets, as increased body temperature has been associated with an increased risk of birth defects.

39

Weight Gain

Weight gain is something which commonly goes along with fibro-myalgia and MPS, and for several reasons. First of all, the pain and stiffness symptoms limit mobility and make exercise difficult, and also the chronic fatigue which is typical of fibromyalgia can make it hard to find the energy to do anything at all. In addition, physical and emotional stresses, which create a metabolic chain reaction, as well as changes in hormonal function, can result in weight gain which, according to one study, amounted to an average of 32 pounds. There is also evidence to suggest that yeast overgrowth, which may contribute to the onset of irritable bowel syndrome, can also lead to sufferers putting on weight.

Some of the medications used to treat fibromyalgia and MPS can, in themselves cause weight gain, while others can increase appetite and so lead to overeating. An increase in the production of the hormone hypocretin, which occurs when an individual experiences a lack of sleep, might also have a part to play. Not only does this lead to an increased state of arousal and fatigue, but also to overeating.

Exercise, as we have described, is a vital part of improving overall health, vitality and fitness and can do much to improve symptoms, but this on its own may not be enough to have much impact on weight gain. Eating a healthy diet which is high in protein and low in carbo-hydrates is also important if you want to try and shift those pounds. Lean meats, eggs, dairy products, tofu and soy meat substitutes are all high in protein, but carbohydrate intake should be limited to fresh fruits and vegetables. In addition, plant and fish oils, almonds and avocados should also be incorporated into the diet. Sugar, bread, pasta, rice, potatoes, carbonated drinks and alcohol, however, should be avoided.

Nutritionists recommend that proteins always be eaten first and that even good carbohydrates should not be eaten by themselves. The reason for this is that when you eat protein first, the protein digestive enzymes in the body are activated and the absorption of carbohydrates slowed down. Another thing to remember is that you need to eat little and often. Aim to eat five or six times a day (either five small meals or three small meals and two larger snacks) or, if you suffer from irritable bowel syndrome, it might be worth trying smaller portions even more frequently. When you do eat, be sure to sit down for your meal rather than eating on the go. Eat slowly, chew well and stop when you feel full but not stuffed.

If the weight gain appears to be associated with the taking of any medications, then do not discontinue use but speak to your doctor to find out whether there might be an alternative that you can use instead. It may be possible, for example, to replace tricyclic antidepressants which are known for causing weight gain, with serotonin selective reuptake inhibitors (SSRIs) which tend to be less problematic in this respect.

Remember that it is always a good idea to check with your health care provider before starting any new diet or exercise programme, so that any other possible causes for weight gain can be ruled out.

40

Travelling

For people suffering from fibromyalgia and/or MPS, the opportunity to get away from it all should be a welcome one, but in some ways it simply raises a number of additional issues. How will you cope with the journey? Will you be able to get out and about and see and do all the things you want to see and do? What happens if you have a flare-up while you are away? Here are some top tips that many sufferers have found particularly helpful.

1. **Rest** – Although it might be enjoyable, travel is also very tiring so be sure to take extra rest before, during and after your holiday. Leave your schedule free for a couple of days before and after travelling so that you have adequate time to store up energy and recover. It is especially important to leave yourself sufficient time after the holiday before going back to work.
2. **Take any medications as scheduled** – Many types of medication work best when they have had the chance to build up in the system, so be sure not to miss any scheduled doses before you go away, whilst you are away and after you get back.
3. **Take your time to prepare** – Rushing around trying to do washing, ironing and packing at the last minute can be both exhausting and stressful. Start well ahead of time and pace yourself.
4. **Plan your itinerary** – When we are away on holiday and there are so many things to see and do, it can often be tempting to overdo things. Do your research in advance and, taking into account what you know yourself to be capable of, plan your itinerary in great detail. Choose those things that you most want to see and do and be sure to fit in periods of inactivity and rest as well. If you are travelling with others who are not aware of your limits, then

discuss these with them in advance and work jointly to come up with a plan which takes your needs into consideration.

Also, make sure that all of your travel arrangements are made well ahead of time, including those for the use of motorised carts or wheelchairs at the airport.

5. **Don't expect too much of yourself** – In just the same way as you have probably had to do in your daily life, it is wise to adjust your expectations for when you are on holiday. You are not going to be able to do as much as you perhaps have done in the past and accepting this fact in advance can help to avoid disappointment. Try to focus on what you can do, rather than what you cannot.

6. **Opt out if you need to** – Even if you had planned to go on excursions or whatever, do not feel afraid to opt out at the last minute if necessary. If you overdo it, you are only likely to cause a flare-up which could see you having to opt out for even longer.

7. **Take frequent breaks during the journey** – Sitting in the same position for hours on end is highly likely to aggravate symptoms, so if you are travelling by car then plan to make regular stops so that you can get out, move around and even do a few stretching exercises. If you are flying, opt for an aisle seat so that you do not have to disturb other passengers when you get up to move around, but do take care that you keep limbs out of the aisle so that you are not bumped. Also, make sure that you have items such as an inflatable pillow, drinking water, snacks and, of course, your medications to hand.

8. **Don't let your pride get in the way** – Many tourist attractions make provision for disabled visitors, such as wheelchairs or motorised carts. Even if you do not normally use these things during your daily life, do not feel too proud to use them while you are away. It could mean the difference between spending the next few days in your hotel room or not.

41

Parenting Issues

Fibromyalgia and MPS are not just adult illnesses but do affect some children and teenagers too. As with the older population of sufferers, females are more commonly affected than males and often the conditions show up during adolescence and between the ages of 13 and 15. In some cases, the conditions present on their own, whilst in others they sit alongside illnesses such as juvenile arthritis. The range of symptoms which are experienced by children, however, is just the same as for adults.

Of course, parenting even a healthy child has its challenges, but parenting one who is constantly in pain and suffering the effects of chronic fatigue, brain fog, irritable bowel syndrome and all the other symptoms which are associated with fibromyalgia and MPS can be particularly demanding, not to mention worrying and stressful. Especially during the time when the doctor is trying to come up with a diagnosis, parents can find themselves feeling frantic in case it turns out that their child has something much more serious or life-threatening. Even after diagnosis, they are understandably anxious about what to expect and about what kind of future their child will have.

Watching for Signs

Fibromyalgia and MPS, as we have seen, are notoriously hard to diagnose and, where children are concerned, there are added complications. With young children in particular, not only may they not be able to communicate what is happening within their bodies, but also they may not appreciate that what they feel is abnormal. If they have experienced pain for as long as they can remember, they are likely to assume that this is a normal state which everyone else simply endures in silence. Even if the pain is identified, however, such as because the child is avoiding certain activities at times, many juvenile illnesses have this symptom in common, so parents need to look out for other signs too.

Of course, one of the main characteristics of both fibromyalgia and MPS is that symptoms tend to come and go, whereas in other illnesses they are generally more consistent. This fact in itself can help to alert parents to the real problem. Sudden and unexplained bouts of overwhelming tiredness, changes in sleeping patterns or spasmodic lapses in concentration, for example, could indicate that your child is suffering from chronic fatigue, a sleep disorder or fibro fog.

Education

Although the treatment of fibromyalgia and MPS in children and teenagers is the same as for adults, where youngsters are concerned it very much needs to involve a team effort. In order for parents and other family members to understand the illnesses and be able to respond appropriately and in the child's best interests, they have to become involved. Without this, not only can there be no semblance of a normal family life, but the child cannot be taught how to live successfully with their condition.

From a practical perspective, you will need to understand any medications which are prescribed for your child and what the side effects of these might be, the exercise regimes that he or she needs to keep up with and how these should be performed, and also how symptoms can be controlled by making adjustments to diet. As well as these things, however, it is essential to understand your role in guiding your child towards living as normal a life as possible. In many ways, changing former habits to improve quality of life is much easier for children to do than for adults though, as most are extremely adaptable and resilient.

Tough Love

Watching a child in pain is an agonising experience and naturally it is one which brings out one's nurturing instincts. For most parents, there is the tendency to want to protect and console, but in the beginning at least, they can be inclined to do so in ways which are ultimately unhelpful. They might, for example, allow their child to take time off school when he or she is tired and in pain, because it simply feels too cruel to insist that they go. By doing so, however, parents risk their youngster becoming dependent and being unable to manage his or her life successfully in the future.

Alongside monitoring the child's condition and playing an active role in ensuring that he or she receives the proper treatment, it is essential that parents provide guidance on how to live with the illness on a daily basis. At times, this may very well involve having to administer some tough love, but without this it is all too easy for children with fibromyalgia or MPS to just give in to their illness and for the whole of their future to be jeopardised. Although there will often be times when living day by day will feel like the easier option, it is essential that parents keep their eyes on the bigger picture and try to make life as normal as possible. If they fail to do so and essentially wrap the child in cotton wool, there is every chance that the life experiences from which they should be learning will be severely limited and that they will find it harder to cope and find happiness later on in life.

As hard as it might sound, children with fibromyalgia or MPS have to be coaxed and sometimes even pushed in the right direction if they are not to use their condition as an excuse for all of the things that they do not want to do in life. Only if they learn to become stronger in themselves will they be able to use the full range of their abilities and meet their full potential.

School Life

As we have said, retaining a sense of normality is important in teaching your child to live with his or her condition and that includes making sure that school life suffers as few interruptions as possible. Just in the same way that an adult sufferer of fibromyalgia or MPS might need to consider certain adaptations to his or her workplace, however, the same may be necessary at school.

Both the pain and the fatigue which are experienced by people with these conditions can mean that things which other children take for granted at school, such as climbing up and down stairs, carrying heavy schoolbags full of books and taking part in physical education classes, can be very difficult. If this is the case, then investigate possibilities such as your child using a lift if one is installed in the building, having a locker or somewhere where books can be stored on each floor to avoid carrying them around and having somewhere quiet where he or she can rest at lunchtimes or during breaks. You may also need to request that your child be excused from physical education lessons if they feel unable to cope with these, but do try to let this be their own decision. If they feel up to it, then let them take part.

Another thing to take into consideration if irritable bowel syndrome or irritable bladder syndrome is an issue is the use of the toilet facilities at school. Some teachers are reluctant to let pupils leave the classroom during lessons to go to the toilet and children typically feel embarrassed about asking. If this is a problem, then speak to the school and try to arrange permission for your child to leave the classroom whenever he or she needs to.

42

Support

Having a chronic condition such as fibromyalgia or MPS can be an intensely frustrating and sometimes lonely experience. Friends, family and work colleagues may not understand what you are going through and even your doctor may not be particularly supportive. Cutting yourself off, however, is not the answer and is only likely to lead to depression and anxiety.

Alongside educating themselves and those around them about their condition, what many patients find particularly helpful is to reach out to fellow sufferers who truly understand their situations. By talking to others through support and self-help groups, they not only feel less alone, but they are also able to pick up a wealth of valuable tips on the strategies that other people have used to cope with and control their illness successfully. To follow, therefore, you will find some of the resources which are available for both online and offline communication.

Support Groups in the UK

A comprehensive list of support groups for fibromyalgia sufferers throughout the UK can be found at **www.ukfibromyalgia.com/ fm-support-groups/fm-support-groups.html**. Simply click on the area of the country that you are interested in to view the contact details of support groups near you.

You can also find a support group directory under the Patient Section at www.fibroaction.org and this site allows you to sign up for a free e-newsletter.

Support Groups in the USA

For readers living in the USA, the website **www.prohealth.com** provides details of local support groups for fibromyalgia sufferers. Click on the link to Community towards the top of the page, select the relevant health topic and identify the state that you live in to view contact details and the website addresses for support groups in your area.

Fibromyalgia and Myofascial Pain Syndrome Organisations

The Fibromyalgia Association UK (**www.fibromyalgia-associationuk.org**) is a UK registered charity which is administered by unpaid volunteers, the majority of whom are sufferers of the condition themselves and work extremely hard to forward the cause of fibromyalgia and raise awareness about the condition. It provides information and support to sufferers and their families, as well as acting as a reference point for medical professionals and operating a national helpline.

In the USA meanwhile, there are several organisations which have been set up both to offer support to sufferers of fibromyalgia and to research the condition. The US National Fibromyalgia Research Association (NFRA) is dedicated to education, treatment and finding a cure for the illness and you can find their website at **www.nfra.net**. The National Fibromyalgia Association (**www.fmaware.org**), meanwhile, is a non-profit organisation which is dedicated to improving the quality of life of sufferers. The American Fibromyalgia Syndrome Association, Inc (AFSA), which can be found online at **www.afsafund.org**, is devoted to funding research which accelerates the pace of medical discoveries with a view to improving the quality of life for patients with fibromyalgia.

Online Support

UK Fibromyalgia, which can be found at www.ukfibromyalgia.com, offers a discussion forum for fibromyalgia sufferers with over 4,000 users. In addition, you can sign up to receive a free e-mail newsletter and subscribe to *FaMily Magazine*. Money raised from the magazine is used to help fund all of the fibromyalgia support groups in the UK and assists them in sourcing necessary small items which are essential to keep them running.

Fibrotalk at **www.fibrotalk.com** is an online support community with forums and chat rooms for sufferers of fibromyalgia. Visitors to the site can view *FOG Magazine* online and free of charge and, by inserting your email address, you can also receive e-news and updates.

Friends International Support is an international online support group which can be found at **www.fms-cfsfriends.com**. With a chat forum and message boards, the site acts as a resource for those suffering from a range of chronic pain conditions rather than just fibromyalgia.

In the USA, **www.prohealth.com** provides message boards and chat rooms for sufferers of a range of different illnesses, including fibromyalgia and irritable bowel syndrome.

Specifically devoted to MPS, the site at **www.dailystrength.org/ c/Myofascial-Pain-Syndrome/support-group** is an online support group where fellow sufferers can discuss relevant topics or can ask questions of an expert.

43

Medico-Legal Implications

As we saw in several of the earlier chapters of this book, both fibro-myalgia and MPS can result from motoring and other types of accidents, with those involving whiplash injuries in particular being believed to be one of the causes of the conditions. In cases where the accident was not the fault of the sufferer, he or she may be able to file a personal injury compensation claim to seek damages from, for example, the other driver in the case of a motoring accident or an employer if the accident was work-related.

Personal Injury Claims

Where individuals have suffered injury or illness as a result of an accident for which they were not responsible, the law permits them to seek damages from the guilty party via the personal injury claims process to compensate them for pain and suffering and to reimburse them for any losses and expenses such as medical fees and any consequent loss of earnings. Generally speaking, any such claim must be made within three years of the accident taking place, although there are certain circumstances when this deadline can be moved, including those where the true nature of the injury did not become apparent until much later.

When making a personal injury claim, you need to be represented by a solicitor. His or her job will be to prove the liability of the other party for your injuries and to persuade the compensator (usually an insurance company) to pay out an appropriate amount of money by way of damages. The job of the legal representative who acts on behalf of the compensator, meanwhile, is to minimise any losses and, if liability is denied, they must provide evidence to support this denial.

Your lawyer will need to show that the onset of fibromyalgia or MPS occurred as a direct result of the other party's negligence, and clearly a suitable medical expert will need to be involved to assess your condition so that the claim can proceed. Once the medical expert's report has been provided to the solicitor, the insurer then has a fixed period of time in which to agree liability and the two sides would then negotiate an appropriate settlement. In most cases where a personal injury claim is successful and liability is accepted, all of the costs associated with the claim will be paid by the other party's insurer.

As you can well imagine, the nature of personal injury claims is that they are adversarial. On the one side, the claimant's solicitor is fighting to achieve an appropriate amount of compensation for his or her client, whose quality of life may have been severely affected as a direct result of an accident which was not their fault. On the other side, the defendant's insurer is fighting his or her corner to avoid any financial liability. In order for a claim to be speedily processed and stand the greatest chance of success, therefore, the expertise of the legal and medical experts who are involved is heavily relied upon.

Burden of Proof

In the world of criminal law, the lawyer for the prosecution must present a case which demonstrates 'beyond reasonable doubt' that the defendant is guilty in order to win. Clearly the case must be absolutely watertight if he or she is to succeed and the work that this involves is, in part, what makes criminal cases so expensive.

Personal injury claims, on the other hand, come under the area of civil law where the burden of proof is on the balance of probabilities. In a case where the plaintiff (the person making the claim) alleges that fibromyalgia or MPS has been the direct result of a road traffic accident, what this means is that, in order to win, the lawyer acting on behalf of the plaintiff simply has to prove that what is alleged by his or her client is, on balance, more likely than what is alleged by the third party who caused the accident.

In the case of illnesses such as fibromyalgia and MPS which are so poorly understood by many doctors, and even less well understood by most solicitors, trying to win a personal injury claim can still be difficult though, and it is for this reason that insurers or solicitors often advise plaintiffs to secure the services of a medico-legal expert who is highly experienced in terms of the injuries sustained to process the claim. In this way, the chances of the claim being successful and damages being paid are much higher.

The Role of a Medico-Legal Expert

Making a personal injury claim clearly involves the need for both legal and medical experts to be involved and the choice of both is crucial in terms of being able to demonstrate that the other party was liable for any injury or illness which resulted from an accident. In the case of medical experts, whilst some have a high degree of knowledge and experience in their particular field of medicine, not all are best equipped to present their evidence in such a way as to be convincing enough to secure the claim. A specialised medico-legal expert, on the other hand, is someone who possesses both the knowledge and skills to make an expert clinical assessment and to present his or her findings in a way that is not only acceptable in a legal sense, but also has the greatest impact in terms of winning the case.

Securing compensation for a personal injury, however, is not the only concern if fibromyalgia or MPS has resulted from an accident. As we have seen throughout the course of this book, being able to return to some semblance of normality in your life involves taking steps to treat and manage the chronic pain and other symptoms which are associated with these conditions. With the right medico-legal expert, individuals can not only ensure that they receive the best possible assessment and diagnosis for legal purposes and so that their claims can be processed quickly, but also the best ongoing medical care from experts in their fields.

Interim Payments

Being diagnosed with fibromyalgia and/or MPS and submitting a personal injury claim is not the end of the story. Immediate costs can arise for treatment and you may already have reached a stage where your earning capability has been affected by your illness. If this is the case, then you may be able to receive part of your compensation in the form of an interim payment after the defendant has admitted liability but in advance of your personal injury case being concluded.

The aim of an interim payment is to alleviate any financial burden which has been caused as a direct result of the accident which caused your illness and it can be used in a variety of ways to help improve your quality of life during the time it takes for a full settlement of your claim to be made. It could, for example, be put towards medical treatment which has already been received or is yet to be received, be used to make any necessary adaptations to your home to make your life easier or to pay for external help or care.

The amount that you can ask for in terms of an interim payment will, of course, depend upon your circumstances, and cannot exceed what would be considered to be a 'reasonable proportion' of the total award that you are likely to receive. You can, however, request more than one interim payment during the course of your claim and, of course, the total amount paid in the interim will be deducted from the overall compensation which is agreed when the case is concluded.

Finding a Personal Injury Solicitor

In most cases involving personal injury, it is not possible to get financial help in the form of legal aid, which means that you could find yourself faced with expensive legal fees which you are unlikely to get back if the case is lost. Nowadays, however, many personal injury solicitors work on a 'no win no fee' basis which, as the name suggests, means that the claimant does not have to pay out for legal fees related to the case unless the case is won and compensation is forthcoming. Even then, if the claim is successful, it is the losing party who picks up the bill for the solicitor's fees and normally for any court fees and medical report costs.

Clearly, for a solicitor to take on a case on a 'no win no fee' basis, he or she must be convinced that your case is likely to be successful, and this is just one of the reasons why it is important to choose a medico-legal expert who can provide you with strong medical evidence.

Medico-Legal Experts' Reports

As we have mentioned, in order to pursue a personal injury claim, your solicitor will need to be provided with a full report of your medical status. Such reports do, of course, vary in detail from medical expert to medical expert, but any good medico-legal service which is multidisciplinary in nature and has access to different expert opinions should be able to provide you with one which is comprehensive and builds a strong case for your claim. At the London Pain Clinic, we provide a full medico-legal report which consists of the following:

1. Details
2. Content
3. Introduction
4. Methodology
5. History
6. Examination
7. Opinion
8. Prognosis
9. Medico-legal declaration
10. Curriculum Vitae

In addition, wherever possible, the report will conclude with our recommendations for treatment.

Conclusion

Fibromyalgia and MPS, if left untreated and unmanaged, can have a devastating effect on the lives of sufferers, but I hope that having read this book you will understand that there is much that can be done to vastly improve your quality of life or that of a sufferer who is close to you.

Understanding something about each of these conditions, the areas of life on which they can have an impact and the range of self-help options and treatments available lies at the very core of being able to carry on a relatively normal life in which pain and other symptoms are minimised. In addition to this, however, finding medical care providers who are not only highly experienced in dealing with similar cases, but who also understand the possible consequences of the illnesses on the lives of patients, is vital.

The potential for chronic illnesses such as fibromyalgia and MPS to take over a sufferer's life are enormous. Being able to remain positive for as much of the time as possible and proactively manage the conditions, however, can mean the difference between sinking into despair and depression or making vast improvements to your quality of life.

Although, as things stand today, the causes of fibromyalgia and MPS are still unknown and there is no cure for either, a great deal of research is still underway. Whilst many general practitioners may not have the time or the opportunity to keep entirely abreast of new findings or revolutionary new treatments, those who work at facilities such as the London Pain Clinic and who specialise in chronic pain conditions such as these are at the cutting edge. In their dealings with literally thousands of patients, their expertise is such that they are able to make a diagnosis much faster, so that an individualised programme of treatment can be developed quickly. In addition, being able to offer a comprehensive range of treatments which tackles the illnesses from all appropriate angles, and having knowledge of the most up-to-date techniques, means that their treatment programmes are far more effective, cutting down the amount of time required to restore patients to acceptable levels of health, as well as associated costs.

Modern treatments for conditions such as fibromyalgia and MPS, such as the use of botox injections, are proving to have a radical effect on the pain symptoms that patients find crippling at times, and yet knowledge of these is generally scant within the medical community as a whole. Despite that, sufferers of chronic pain conditions would never dream of entrusting other aspects of their lives to anybody other than a specialist expert, however, many do still rely on the help of generalists when it comes to their health – and often pay the price in terms of extended waiting times for their illness to be diagnosed and treated effectively.

As I have talked about in the final chapter of this book, another area where those with fibromyalgia and/or MPS frequently miss opportunities to improve their quality of life is in relation to compensation for the onset of their illness where this was caused by a third party. In many cases, having been diagnosed with either of these conditions, patients are financially unable to seek out the very best and most effective treatment. Armed with expert medical and legal representation, however, they could have access to funds which could improve their lives dramatically.

For all of the bad news that a diagnosis of fibromyalgia or MPS might bring, there is a bright side. You are certainly not alone and there is certainly no reason why your life needs to continue to be one which is filled with pain and misery. Whilst we hope that there is a cure just waiting to be found around the next corner, in the meantime you can take control and you can learn to live a successful and happy life even with your condition.

So, all it remains for me to say is that I hope this book has been of some benefit to you and that it has provided you with a greater insight into your options and inspired in you a greater sense of hope for your future. If there is any further information, advice or support that I can offer which might help you to work towards improving your condition and your quality of life, then please don't hesitate to contact me.

All the best!

Dr Christopher Jenner MB BS, FCRA
London Pain Clinic
www.londonpainclinic.com

Index